THE COMPLETE GUIDE TO
STRENGTH TRAINING

Fifth edition

Anita Bean

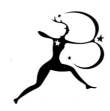

Bloomsbury Sport
An imprint of Bloomsbury Publishing Plc

50 Bedford Square
London
WC1B 3DP
UK

1385 Broadway
New York
NY 10018
USA

www.bloomsbury.com

BLOOMSBURY and the Diana logo are trademarks of Bloomsbury Publishing Plc

First edition published 1997, second edition 2001, third edition 2005, fourth edition 2008.
This fifth edition published 2015.

© Anita Bean, 2015
Cover image © Getty Images

Anita Bean has asserted her right under the Copyright, Designs and Patents Act, 1988,
to be identified as Author of this work.

All rights reserved. No part of this publication may be reproduced or transmitted in any
form or by any means, electronic or mechanical, including photocopying, recording, or any
information storage or retrieval system, without prior permission in writing from
the publishers.

No responsibility for loss caused to any individual or organization acting on or refraining
from action as a result of the material in this publication can be accepted by Bloomsbury
or the author.

British Library Cataloguing-in-Publication Data
A catalogue record for this book is available from the British Library.

ISBN: PB: 978-1-4729-1065-3
ePDF: 978-1-4729-1063-9
ePub: 978-1-4729-1062-2

2 4 6 8 10 9 7 5 3 1

Typeset in 10.75pt on 14pt Adobe Caslon by Margaret Brain, Wisbech, Cambs
Printed and bound in China by Toppan Leefung Printing

Bloomsbury Publishing Plc makes every effort to ensure that the papers used in the
manufacture of our books are natural, recyclable products made from wood grown in
well-managed forests. Our manufacturing processes conform to the environmental
regulations of the country of origin.

To find out more about our authors and books visit www.bloomsbury.com. Here you will
find extracts, author interviews, details of forthcoming events and the option to sign up
for our newsletters.

CONTENTS

List of abbreviations		5
Acknowledgements		5
Foreword		6
Preface to the fifth edition		7
PART ONE	MUSCLE SCIENCE	**8**
Chapter 1	Introduction	10
Chapter 2	Principles of muscle growth	14
Chapter 3	Principles and methods of strength training	23
Chapter 4	Programme design	36
Chapter 5	How to get started	46
Chapter 6	Warming up	56
PART TWO	NUTRITION	**58**
Chapter 7	Build muscle not fat	60
Chapter 8	Sports supplements	85
PART THREE	THE EXERCISES	**100**
Chapter 9	The lower body	104
Chapter 10	The back	120
Chapter 11	The chest	132

Chapter 12	The shoulders	142
Chapter 13	The arms	151
Chapter 14	The abdominals	163
Chapter 15	Body weight exercises	180
Chapter 16	Power/plyometric exercises	189
Chapter 17	The stretches	201
PART FOUR	TRAINING PROGRAMMES	**208**
Chapter 18	The beginner's programme	210
Chapter 19	The intermediate's programme	217
Chapter 20	The advanced programme	223
Chapter 21	The strength programme	230
Chapter 22	Body weight workouts	232
Chapter 23	Power workouts	234
Chapter 24	Training for sports programmes	236
Chapter 25	The cardiovascular programme	246
Chapter 26	Training for specific results	253
Appendix		265
References		271
Further reading		280
Glossary		281
Index		283

List of Abbreviations

1RM	One-rep max	**GH**	Growth hormone
ATP	Adenosine triphosphate	**HR**	Heart rate
bpm	Beats per minute	**EAAs**	Essential amino acids
BV	Biological value	**MHR**	Maximum heart rate
BCAAs	Branched chained amino acids	**MRP**	Meal replacement product
DAAs	Dispensable amino acids	**ORAC**	Oxygen Radical Absorbance Capacity
DHA	Docosahexaenoic acid	**PC**	Phosphocreatine
DPA	Docosapentaenoic acid	**ROM**	Range of movement
EPA	Eicosapentaenoic acid	**RPE**	Rating of perceived exertion
EPOC	Excess post-exercise oxygen consumption	**RDA**	Recommended daily amount
FT	Fast twitch	**Reps**	Repetitions
GLA	Gamma-linolenic acid	**RMR**	Resting metabolic rate
GI	Glycaemic index	**ST**	Slow twitch
GTOs	Golgi tendon organs	**THR**	Training heart rate

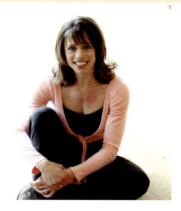

ACKNOWLEDGEMENTS

I have been most fortunate to work with many great strength athletes and coaches over the years and would like to thank them for their knowledge and encouragement to write this book. In particular, I would like to thank Professor Andrew Jones for his insights, personal trainers James Matthews, Alice Tourell and Rachel Anne Hobbs for their proficiency demonstrating the exercises, photographer and artist Tom Croft for his creativity and Surrey Sports Park for use of the gym. As always, I am very grateful to my husband, Simon, for his unerring patience, my daughters Chloe and Lucy, now accomplished athletes, for providing enormous inspiration for this 5th edition. And finally, I would like to thank my commissioning editor Charlotte Croft and the wonderful team at Bloomsbury Sport for all their support and hard work making this book possible.

Anita Bean

FOREWORD

Strength training, in all its forms, is now widely acknowledged as being an essential component of any overall fitness training programme. This is true whether the goal is to develop musculo-skeletal health, to maintain function in older age, or to maximise performance in competitive sport.

In my younger days, as an international distance runner, I included strength training in my overall programme because I intuitively felt that it helped my performance. Interestingly, recent research has confirmed that indeed this is the case, and today's athletes complete sophisticated resistance training regimens as an integral part of their preparation for competition. Although I no longer compete, I continue a balanced exercise programme but with a much greater emphasis on resistance training in an attempt to limit the extent of sarcopenia (loss of muscle mass commencing in middle age). Again, research now strongly indicates that the maintenance of muscle mass is essential in the maintenance of function and independence in older age.

This 5th edition of *The Complete Guide to Strength Training* is a must-read for anyone interested in the benefits of resistance training for health and performance. The advice is comprehensive, totally up-to-date, based on the latest scientific evidence and beautifully illustrated. The book provides state-of-the-art recommendations for the development of strength, power, and muscular hypertrophy, and encompasses training techniques involving free weights, body-weight exercises and plyometrics. Importantly, it also provides expert advice on appropriate nutrition and supplementation to support strength training, whether the goal is to build muscle or to lose body fat. Overall, I recommend this book as an essential companion for anyone – younger or older, and whether of high or low present fitness – wishing to reap the benefits of regular strength training.

Andrew M Jones PhD
Professor of Applied Physiology
The University of Exeter

PREFACE TO THE FIFTH EDITION

I wrote the first edition of *The Complete Guide to Strength Training* in 1997 as a tribute to my success as a natural bodybuilding champion (EFBB British Lightweight Champion, 1991) and to encapsulate the fulfilment I had experienced from 15 years of strength training. I wanted to share with you my professional knowledge as a nutritionist and fitness instructor, as well as my first-hand experience as a competitor. I am passionate about training and believe everyone can benefit from it, both physically and mentally.

This book translates the current science of training and nutrition into practical advice. It provides you with an integrated plan of action to achieve your training goals. I have drawn together scientifically proven training methods and cutting-edge nutritional advice to devise training programmes for beginners, intermediates and advanced trainers.

Part One of this book explains the principles of strength training, muscle growth and training methods. Part Two covers nutrition and sports supplements as well as sample menu plans for muscle gain. Part Three provides an illustrated, step-by-step guide to the exercises included in the training programmes, with comprehensive training technique tips. All this information is consolidated in the training programmes presented in Part Four, where I have devised detailed week-by-week workouts for beginners, intermediates and advanced trainers, as well as workouts for different sports. Throughout the text I have included references to the original sources of information, giving you the opportunity to delve further into particular topics if you wish.

This updated fifth edition includes cutting-edge information on nutrition and sports supplements, new exercises, and additional programmes for increasing strength, muscle and explosive power, body weight workouts and plyometric training.

Since the publication of the first edition I have received many emails from people who have followed the training programmes in this book with amazing results. Some people have gained impressive amounts of muscle weight and/or lost body fat, others have benefited from the extra strength needed for other sports, while others have been inspired to follow a healthier and fitter lifestyle. Whatever your goals, I sincerely hope you, too, benefit from the advice given in this book.

Although I no longer compete in bodybuilding, I continue training regularly – albeit with considerably lighter weights than previously. I also practise yoga daily for the physical, mental and spiritual benefits it gives me. Physical fitness and good health are our most valuable assets and I am grateful to have the opportunity to share my knowledge and experience with you. I wish you every success in achieving your own training goals, and hope you enjoy reaping the rewards.

Anita Bean

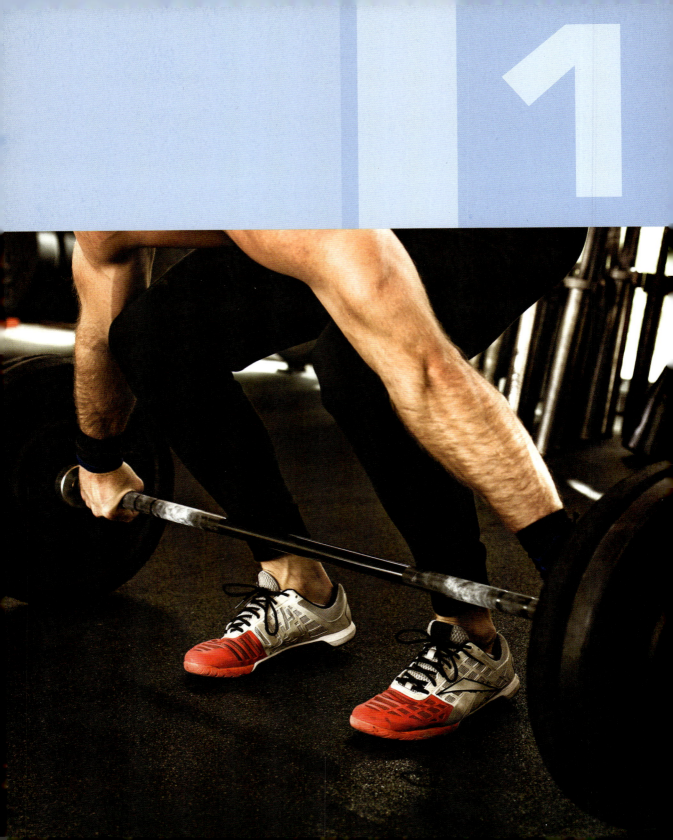

PART **ONE**

MUSCLE SCIENCE

A stronger, leaner, fitter body is within your grasp. By picking up this book, you've made a commitment to change. Whether you want to tone up, develop muscle size or improve your performance in sport, this book will help you achieve your goals. But first, a good understanding of how your muscles work, how they grow and the various training methods will enable you to target your training more effectively. The following chapters equip you with the training know-how you need to get started on the road to success.

BENEFITS OF STRENGTH TRAINING

Strength training is not only about lifting weights and building muscle, it's also about creating a balanced musculature that can move with grace and fluidity, respond optimally to any physical demand, perform well in sport, minimise injury risk and – importantly – be aesthetically pleasing. Training with weights also develops your inner strength, gives you a terrific sense of accomplishment, builds confidence and fosters a positive mental attitude.

INCREASED MUSCLE MASS AND STRENGTH

A well-planned resistance training programme increases muscle size and strength. In contrast, endurance activities do not produce significant changes in strength or muscle mass. Research has shown that a basic resistance training programme lasting just 25 minutes, 3 times a week, can increase muscle mass by about 1 kg over an 8-week period (Campbell *et al*, 1994), while lean mass gains of 20 per cent of your starting body weight are common after the first year of training. According to a review of studies, 10 weeks of resistance training may increase lean weight by 1.4 kg, increase resting metabolic rate by 7 per cent, and reduce fat weight by 1.8 kg (Westcott, 2012).

STRONGER TENDONS AND LIGAMENTS

Resistance training increases the strength of the tendons and ligaments, and therefore improves joint stability. It stimulates the production of collagen proteins in the tendons and ligaments (Campbell *et al*, 1994), causing an increase in their structural strength.

INCREASED METABOLIC RATE

Strength training increases the resting metabolic rate (RMR) – the rate at which your body burns calories – by increasing muscle mass. Muscle has a higher energy requirement than fat tissue, so the more muscle you have, the higher your metabolic rate.

At rest, 0.45 kg (1 lb) of muscle tissue burns approximately 6 kcal/day, compared with fat which burns 2–4 kcal per 0.45 kg (1 lb) (Wang *et al*, 2011). Adding muscle increases your RMR and total daily calorie expenditure. One study found that 1.4 kg of extra muscle increases RMR by 7 per cent and daily calorie requirement by 15 per cent (Forbes, 1976). During exercise, energy expenditure rises dramatically – 5 to 10 times above the resting level. Thus, the more muscle tissue you have, the greater the number of calories expended during exercise and at rest.

ANTI-AGEING BENEFITS

Without exercise, adults typically experience a 2–5 per cent decrease in their metabolic rate and an increase of 7 kg of fat every decade (Wolfe, 2006; Evans & Rosenberg, 1992). This is due largely to a loss of muscle tissue and may translate into unwanted body fat gain. Without strength training, adults typically lose 3–8 per cent of muscle mass every decade from the age of 30 (Flack et al, 2011) and 5–10 per cent afer the age of 50 (Marcell, 2003). Muscle loss occurs mainly in the fast-twitch (FT) muscle fibres, which are involved in strength and explosive activities (see p. 189). This cannot be prevented by cardiovascular exercise – only strength training maintains muscle mass and strength as you get older. Therefore, strength training is an excellent way of preserving muscle mass, preventing a reduction of metabolic rate, and avoiding fat gain with age.

REDUCED BODY FAT

Strength training can help reduce body fat by increasing the metabolic rate and therefore daily calorie expenditure. One study found that although aerobic training produced greater weight loss, strength training in combination with aerobic training resulted in greater fat loss and muscle gain, i.e. an improved body composition, compared with those doing aerobic training only (Willis et al, 2012). A review of 15 randomised controlled trials also concluded that a combined programme of strength and aerobic training is more effective for reducing body fat than aerobic training or strength training only (Schwingshackl et al, 2013).

INCREASED BONE DENSITY

Strength training improves bone strength, and increases bone protein and mineral content (Hurley, 1994). Studies show that the bones under the most stress from resistance training have the highest bone mineral content (Taafe et al, 1997). For example, it has been shown that there are significant increases in the bone mineral content of the upper femur (thigh) after 4 months of strength training (Menkes et al, 1993). The ACSM recommend 2–3 weekly sessions of resistance training to preserve bone mass (Kohrt et al, 2004).

REDUCED BLOOD PRESSURE

Strength training has been shown to lower both systolic and diastolic blood pressure. The effect is even greater if strength training is combined with aerobic exercise. One study of 15 men with high blood pressure found that 12 weeks of strength training (3 times a week) resulted in a decrease in systolic blood pressure of 16 mm Hg, and diastolic blood pressure of 12 mm Hg ('mm Hg' stands for 'mm of mercury', which is the standard unit of measurement for blood pressure) (Moraes et al, 2012).

REDUCED BLOOD CHOLESTEROL AND BLOOD FATS

Studies have demonstrated improvements in blood cholesterol and blood triglycerides (fats) through several weeks of strength training (Hurley, 1994; Stone et al, 1982).

IMPROVED POSTURE

Strength training greatly improves overall posture, as well as correcting specific postural faults. A number of factors influence our posture, including skeletal structure, basic body type, strength and flexibility. Obviously, the first and second factors are controlled by our genetic make-up and cannot be altered. However, strength and flexibility can be changed through training or disuse (i.e. increased or decreased demand). Imbalances in these two components lead to postural faults, but these may be corrected through specific strength training exercises and stretches.

INJURY PREVENTION

A well-conditioned and well-balanced musculo-skeletal system has a much smaller chance of sustaining injury. A stronger body is better able to avoid or resist impact injuries from falls and activities such as running or jumping. Muscular imbalances are a common cause of injury: for example, underdeveloped hamstrings (back of the thighs) relative to the quadriceps (front of the thighs) can make the knee joint unstable, thus increasing injury risk.

The majority of lower-back problems are due to weakness or imbalance of the deep muscles close to the spine and pelvis, which contribute to core stability. A well-designed strength training programme will improve the strength of the trunk stabilisers – the transverse abdominis and the lumbar multifidus – thus reducing the likelihood of injury. One study found that patients suffering lower-back pain had significantly less pain after 10 weeks of specific strength exercises (Risch *et al*, 1993).

IMPROVED PSYCHOLOGICAL WELL-BEING

Consistent strength training helps to reduce stress, anxiety and depression, uplift your mood, and promote more restful sleep. It may help decrease muscle tension due to the intensity of the muscular contractions. It also improves body image, which has a major effect on psychological well-being. Participants report that they have more energy, greater confidence and are prouder of their appearance.

IMPROVED APPEARANCE

Personal appearance is greatly improved by strength training due to increased muscle tone, strength, function and improved posture. Changes in body composition mean an increase in lean mass and decrease in fat mass, both of which enhance the way you look.

STRENGTH TRAINING MYTHS

Despite the well-recognised benefits of strength training discussed above, there are many myths that still exist.

MYTH 1: STRENGTH TRAINING MAKES WOMEN TOO BULKY

Some women avoid strength training for fear of looking too masculine. However, strength training actually enhances a woman's femininity; it improves muscle tone and definition, and creates a better body shape. Increases in muscle mass can be made, but women can never achieve the muscle bulk of men. This is due to the fact that men have 10 times as much of the muscle-building hormone, testosterone, in their systems.

Women are, therefore, genetically programmed not to achieve the muscle bulk of men.

MYTH 2: IF YOU STOP TRAINING, MUSCLE TURNS TO FAT

It is impossible for muscle to turn to fat, as it is a completely different type of body tissue. Muscle mass and strength will gradually decrease if you stop training (some physiologists believe that a muscle will never quite return to its pre-training state), and fat stores will increase if you eat more calories than you need over a period of time. However, one will not turn into the other! Once a certain muscle mass has been achieved through regular strength training, this can be maintained by training less frequently (once or twice a week).

MYTH 3: STRENGTH TRAINING MAKES YOU MUSCLE-BOUND AND DECREASES FLEXIBILITY

Increasing your muscle mass does not make you muscle-bound, reduce your flexibility or reduce your speed in athletic activities. On the contrary, if you train correctly – performing each exercise in strict form through a full range of motion (ROM) that gives your muscles and joints a full stretch – you can maintain and even improve flexibility. Your ROM may decrease when you lift heavy weights, so compensate for this by doing full ROM stretches between sets and especially at the end of your workout.

Continued use of heavier weights, partial repetitions and performing exercises with an incomplete ROM ('cheating reps') usually results in reduced flexibility. Also, if you have one muscle group (e.g. the quadriceps) that is over-developed in comparison with the opposing group (e.g. the hamstrings), this can cause reduced flexibility in that opposing muscle group. This is common in cyclists and footballers due to the larger volume of work performed by the quadriceps. In any case, stretching the relevant muscles after training will help prevent them shortening and increase their flexibility.

It has been demonstrated that a strong muscle can contract more quickly and generate more power than a weak one. In fact, the physiques of world-class sprinters are very muscular, which shows that increased muscle mass does not hinder your speed or flexibility.

MYTH 4: STRENGTH TRAINING HARMS THE JOINTS

When performed properly and safely, strength training improves the strength of the ligaments that hold a joint together, thus making the joint more stable and less prone to injury. Impact movements such as running and jumping can unduly stress the ligaments and make the joints more susceptible to injury. The controlled, no-impact movements used in strength training, however, place far less stress on the joints than most other forms of exercise, so are a good way of strengthening them.

PRINCIPLES OF MUSCLE GROWTH

How do muscles get bigger? If you lift weights, eat and rest, your muscles grow. True, but the science behind it all goes much deeper. This chapter tells you how muscles are made up, how they work and how they get bigger. The more you know, the more easily you will reach your training goals.

MUSCLE FITNESS

Strength training can develop three components of muscle fitness: strength, endurance and power. The amount of weight lifted, the speed of movement and the number of repetitions will determine which aspect is developed most. In general, using heavy weights for a lower number of repetitions (fewer than 12) develops strength and size; using lighter weights for a higher number of repetitions develops endurance; explosive movements develop power.

MUSCULAR STRENGTH

Muscular strength is the amount of force a muscle can produce – for example, the amount of weight that can be lifted. This is developed by heavy weights. Generally, the larger the muscle, the stronger it is, although other factors such as neuromuscular adaptation (the number of fibres controlled and recruited by your nervous system) also affect your strength.

MUSCULAR ENDURANCE

Muscular endurance is the ability of a muscle to continue contracting against a resistance. This is developed by maintaining a constant workload for increasing periods of time – lifting a weight for 12 or more repetitions then building up to, say, 15, 20 and so on, as endurance improves. Long-distance cycling will develop muscle endurance in the thigh muscles, for example.

MUSCULAR POWER

Muscular power is the ability to produce both strength and speed. It involves generating a great force as rapidly as possible and is therefore characterised by explosive movements. It is developed by lifting near maximal weights (a weight heavy enough to allow 1–5 repetitions) very rapidly (see p. 189) and is an important aspect of performance for most sports.

MUSCLE ACTIONS

CONCENTRIC MUSCLE ACTIONS

These occur when a muscle shortens during contraction. Examples of concentric actions include the upward phase of a biceps curl and the upward phase of a bench press.

ECCENTRIC MUSCLE ACTIONS

These are the reverse of a concentric action – they return the muscle to its original starting point. The muscle lengthens as the joint angle increases, releasing under controlled tension. Examples of eccentric actions include the downward phase of a biceps curl and the lowering phase of a bench press.

ISOMETRIC MUSCLE ACTIONS

These occur when the muscle develops tension without changing its length. For example, an isometric contraction develops during a biceps curl if you cannot continue the movement beyond the midpoint – the tension in your biceps equals the resistance of the barbell.

PRIME MOVER/AGONIST

The muscle that brings about a movement is called the *prime mover* or agonist. For example, during a biceps curl, the prime mover is the biceps muscle.

ANTAGONIST

The muscle that acts in opposition to the prime mover, which may slow it down or stop the movement, is called the *antagonist*. It helps to keep the joint stable and during most movements it is relaxed, allowing the movement to be performed efficiently. For example, during a biceps curl the triceps acts as the antagonist and needs to be relaxed to allow the arm to be flexed smoothly.

MUSCLE STRUCTURE

Muscles make up about 45 per cent of your body's weight. They are 80 per cent water; the rest is mostly protein. Each muscle is made up of cylindrical fibres (sometimes called muscle cells), which are about 50–100 micrometres in diameter (the width of a human hair). They range from a few centimetres in length to 1 m, and can run the entire length of the muscle. These fibres are grouped in bundles called fasciculi, each separately wrapped in a sheath (perimysium) that holds them together.

Each muscle fibre comprises thread-like strands called myofibrils, each of which is about 1 micrometre in diameter, or $\frac{1}{100}$th the diameter of a human hair. These hold myofilaments containing the contractile proteins myosin (thick filaments) and actin (thin filaments), whose actions are responsible for muscle contraction (see Figure 2.1). To a large extent, your muscle's

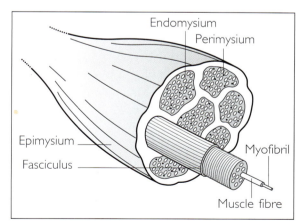

Figure 2.1 The structure of skeletal muscle

cross-sectional area, together with the number and length of its fibres, determine its strength. You cannot change the number of fibres in your muscle, but you can increase both its cross-sectional areas through strength training, and the number of muscle fibres recruited when executing any given movement.

SYNERGIST

A muscle that assists indirectly in a movement is called a *synergist*. For example, in a biceps curl the muscles of the forearm act as synergists because they cross the elbow joint and help to bring about the movement.

MUSCLE FIBRE TYPES

Your muscle fibres can be divided into two types:

1. slow-twitch (ST), or type I, fibres
2. fast-twitch (FT), or type II, fibres.

ST fibres are used for endurance activities. They contract relatively slowly, produce less tension and prefer to use oxygen to produce energy (i.e. aerobic metabolism). They have many capillaries and mitochondria (the powerhouses of cells) and can easily make use of both fat and carbohydrate for fuel. ST fibres do not tire easily so are used for low-intensity, long-duration aerobic activities such as walking and jogging.

FT fibres are essentially the opposite. They are best suited to anaerobic activities – anything requiring more than 25 per cent of your maximum strength. These fibres can generate high levels of tension, contract very rapidly but have poor endurance.

FT fibres can be further subdivided into FTa (type IIa) and FTb (type IIb) fibres, based on their ability to produce energy under aerobic conditions. FTa fibres have more capillaries surrounding them, more mitochondria and a greater number of aerobic enzymes than FTb fibres and, therefore, are more resistant to fatigue. The FTb fibres have the highest anaerobic capacity but the lowest endurance capacity of all fibre types. They tire very quickly and are used almost exclusively for explosive power activities such as sprinting and jumping.

Each muscle has a mix of FT and ST fibres, and this mix is largely genetically determined. Whether a muscle fibre is FT or ST is determined before birth and in the first few years of life. After this time there is little you can do to change the number or structure of your muscle fibres. Some people are born with a predominance

Can you change your muscle fibres?

It is possible to change the function of certain muscle fibre types through specific kinds of training. With aerobic training, FTa fibres can learn to use more oxygen and so assume some of the characteristics of ST fibres – i.e. they become more aerobic – while FTb fibres begin to assume some of the characteristics of FTa fibres and gain greater endurance. So, endurance training does not change the fibre type but will increase the muscles' aerobic capacity. It is not, however, possible for changes to occur in the opposite direction – i.e. for ST fibres to assume the characteristics of FT fibres.

of FT fibres, which makes them better suited to activities requiring speed, strength or power.

Put simply, a top sprinter or weightlifter would probably have a high percentage of explosive FT fibres and fewer ST fibres, while an endurance athlete is more likely to have a high percentage of ST fibres and fewer FT fibres.

Regardless of your genetically determined fibre mix, you can still increase muscle size and strength through intensive training and good nutrition.

MUSCLE FIBRES AND STRENGTH TRAINING

When you lift light weights – for example, during your warm-up sets or during a weight training circuit – your ST fibres carry out most of the work. As you increase the weight lifted, an increasing number of FTa and FTb fibres are also recruited. When you lift very heavy or maximal weights, both ST and FTa fibres, and virtually all of the FTb fibres, are recruited. The recruitment of different fibre types as the intensity of exercise (i.e. weight lifted) increases is shown in Figure 2.2.

So, if you perform mostly light, high-repetition training, you will stimulate mostly ST fibres and develop good muscular endurance but limited strength and size. If you incorporate both medium and low-repetition training (i.e. using moderate and heavy weights) into your programme (bodybuilding), you will stimulate all three fibre types and therefore develop good strength, size and muscular endurance. If you perform only heavy, low-repetition training (maximal strength training), you will mainly stimulate the FTb fibres and develop good strength and moderate size, but poor muscular endurance.

Why do some people gain strength and muscle size more easily than others?
One explanation is that they have a greater number of muscle fibres in each motor unit. The number of fibres per motor unit is genetically determined and varies between 20 and 500, but averages around 200. So, if you have above-average fibre numbers in each motor unit, you can generate a greater force output compared to the average person. This creates a bigger stimulus for muscle growth, so your gains in strength and size will be faster.

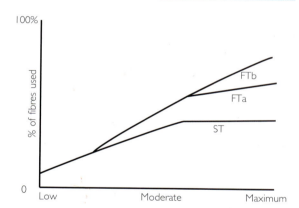

Figure 2.2 The recruitment of ST and FT muscle fibres

The all or nothing principle – A muscle fibre either contracts or it doesn't and, when it does, it contracts with maximal force.
The size principle – As training load increases, progressively more muscle fibres are activated.

HOW MUSCLES WORK

Your muscles are connected to your nervous system. They are fired, or activated, by motor nerves, and a single motor nerve may stimulate anywhere between one and several hundred muscle fibres. A nerve cell and a muscle fibre are called a motor unit. When a motor nerve is stimulated it causes all of the muscle fibres to contract. This is the all or nothing principle (see box).

The number of motor units involved in a contraction depends on the load imposed on the muscle. With a light load (weight), only a few motor units – those activating the ST fibres – are pulled into action. As the load increases, progressively more motor units will be recruited – activating the FT fibres – until, with a maximal weight, all (or almost all) of the motor units will be recruited. Therefore, to stimulate the whole muscle, you have to work with weights that require an all-out effort. Otherwise, the highest threshold motor units never get recruited.

Muscle contraction can be explained by the sliding filament theory of muscle contraction. This involves the two contractile proteins, actin and myosin. When an impulse from a motor nerve reaches the muscle fibre, it creates chemical changes that cause the actin filaments to slide inwards on the myosin filaments. The myosin filaments contain cross-bridges – which are tiny extensions that reach towards the actin filaments. The myosin binds to the actin via these cross-bridges, causing them to swivel and pull the myosin filaments over the actin filaments (see Figure 2.3). This sliding is what causes the muscle to shorten and thicken – or contract. Once the stimulation stops, the actin and myosin filaments move apart and the muscle returns to its resting length and thickness.

The force generated by the muscle depends on the weight lifted and its original length before contraction. If it is in its normal resting length, or slightly longer (slightly stretched), all of the cross-bridges on the myosin can connect with the actin filaments, creating greater force. For example, during a biceps curl, you will generate maximal force in the biceps muscle by starting with your arms in the fully straightened position. Starting with your arms slightly flexed will reduce the force developed and therefore the training stimulus, irrespective of the weight lifted.

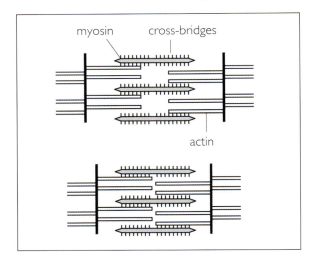

Figure 2.3 Contraction of skeletal muscle

HOW MUSCLES GROW

Increases in strength are the combined result of changes in the way nerve pathways serve the motor units – neuromuscular adaptations – and developing bigger muscles – hypertrophy.

When you begin lifting weights, most of the strength gains come from the nerves controlling the muscle-firing pattern becoming more efficient. The nervous system adapts to a progressive overload by improving its ability to recruit additional muscle fibres and generate more force. The greater the number of motor units involved, the greater the force of contraction. In fact, your strength gains during the first 6–8 weeks of starting a strength training programme are due mostly to neuromuscular adaptation. Don't be put off if you don't get bigger muscles after the first couple of months of training. Your nervous system adapts to the new stimulus first, allowing you to maximise your strength with the muscle you already have. This is called neuromuscular adaptation.

After this initial period, your muscles start to grow in size and this contributes to your strength gains. The repeated contraction of muscles during resistance training causes damage in the muscle tissue. The muscle proteins (actin and myosin) undergo micro-trauma – microscopic tears occur in the muscle fibres and connective tissue. This occurs primarily during the eccentric phase of the motion (see p. 15) and causes the soreness you feel for a few days after an intense workout. During the rest period between workouts, new proteins are built up, the connective tissue is repaired, the muscle fibres enlarge, and the muscle increases in diameter and strength.

The increase in muscle size – hypertrophy – is due to an increase in the cross-sectional area of the individual fibres, rather than an increase in the number of fibres (hyperplasia) (Goldberg *et al*, 1975; Macdougall *et al*, 1994; Sale *et al*, 1987). This is the result of an increase in actin and myosin, and an increase in the number of filaments within the fibres (Macdougall *et al*, 1980). The new filaments are added in layers to the outside of the existing bundles of filaments. Thus each muscle fibre becomes denser and bigger, enlarging the whole muscle and increasing its strength.

The FT fibres increase in size more readily and at a faster rate than ST fibres (Schmidtbleicher & Haralambie, 1981). Therefore, it is the growth of FT fibres that results in an increase in muscle mass and strength (Dons *et al*, 1979).

Lifting weights also causes an increase in the number of blood vessels in the muscle. This means that more oxygen, fuel and nutrients can be delivered to the muscles, and metabolic waste products can be removed more readily. The overall result is one of increased efficiency, strength and size.

The attached tendons, ligaments and bones also increase in strength, and so the whole surrounding structural framework becomes stronger.

Hypertrophy

Training forces your muscles to do more work than normal to overcome the load. This process is called overloading and leads to increases in muscle strength and size through a process called hypertrophy.

Neuromuscular adaptation

Changes in the way nerve pathways serve the motor units are called neuromuscular adaptation. It's a type of motor learning – your body learns to assign more and more motor units to the movements and so you get stronger.

Another key factor in muscle growth is improved coordination. The ability to coordinate specific movements can only be learned through practice. To perform an efficient lift, you need to relax the antagonistic muscles, so that unnecessary movement does not affect the force of the prime movers (see below). A well-coordinated group of muscles will be able to achieve a greater training effect and, therefore, better strength gains.

Muscle tone

Muscle tone refers to the relative state of contraction during rest. When you begin training, there is an increase in muscle tone – your muscles feel tighter – due to an increase in the packing density of the filaments.

The muscle becomes stronger and firmer to the touch in the relaxed state. This is what is commonly called 'good muscle tone'. If you don't increase your training level but maintain the same volume, the muscles do not continue to adapt so you will simply stay toned and will not increase in size. If you were to increase your training level (i.e. training volume and intensity), your muscles would increase in size as well as density.

FACTORS AFFECTING MUSCLE MASS

The amount of muscle mass you can expect to gain will be determined by your genetic make-up, your training programme and your diet. You cannot change your genes, but by understanding your personal limitations you can work out your real strengths and weaknesses and set realistic goals. The following four factors will help you to decide your natural potential for muscle growth.

1. BODY TYPE

Your body type dictates your genetic potential to add muscle or fat (see p. 253). If you have a naturally slender frame with a small musculature (ectomorphic body type), your muscle gains will be slower and, ultimately, smaller than someone with a naturally athletic frame (mesomorphic body type). Chances are you will never closely resemble a heavyweight bodybuilder but, with hard work in the gym, you could achieve more of a lifeguard's physique. If you have a naturally large, stocky frame with a fair amount of body fat (endomorphic body type), you will gain muscle readily but will need to work harder with your cardiovascular training and cut back your calorie intake in order for your muscles to show. You may not achieve the sharp definition of a world-class 100 m sprinter but you could achieve the impressive muscle bulk and athleticism of a rugby player. If you are fortunate enough to be blessed with broad shoulders, narrow waist and hips and low body fat (mesomorph), you could achieve the perfect symmetry of a champion bodybuilder!

2. MUSCLE FIBRE MIX

You probably have a rough idea of your mix of fast-twitch (FT) and slow-twitch (ST) muscle fibres from your natural sporting ability. If you tend to do well at sports requiring a lot of strength, speed and power, you probably have a high ratio of FT to ST fibres and will tend to gain muscle size relatively fast. On the other hand, if you tend to perform better in endurance activities, you probably have a higher proportion of ST fibres and will make slower muscle size gains. Since FT muscle fibres have the highest capacity for hypertrophy, you will experience greater gains if you have a high proportion of these.

3. MOTOR UNITS

The arrangement of your motor units – the number of muscle fibres activated by each motor nerve – determines your rate of progress too. People who tend to gain strength and size very rapidly probably have an above-average number of muscle fibres in each motor unit. For the same effort, they generate a higher force output than the average person. This creates a bigger stimulus for muscle growth.

4. HORMONAL BALANCE

Your natural hormonal balance will affect your degree of muscularity and how fast you can add muscle. If you have naturally high levels of anabolic hormones such as testosterone and growth hormone (GH), you will respond to a strength training programme more readily, and achieve greater gains in muscle mass and strength than more average people. This explains why women generally never achieve the muscle bulk and strength of men, despite heavy training, as they have only one-tenth of the testosterone levels. Only by taking anabolic steroids can they achieve more masculine proportions.

THE BOTTOM LINE

Even if you have few of these genetically determined factors on your side, you can still make great gains by paying extra attention to the quality of your training and your eating plan. Regardless of your body type, muscle fibre-type mix, motor unit make-up and hormonal level, you can improve your physique beyond measure by following a well-planned training and nutrition programme.

HOW FAST CAN I EXPECT TO GAIN WEIGHT?

Most men can expect to gain 0.5–1 kg/month on an established programme (ACSM, 2009; Houston, 1999). Women usually experience about 50–75 per cent of the gains of men – i.e. 0.25–0.75 kg/month – partly due to their smaller initial body weight and smaller muscle mass, and partly due to lower levels of anabolic hormones. Your weight gain may be as much as 2 kg/month during the first few months of starting strength training. In fact, lean mass gains of 20 per cent of your starting body weight are common after the first year of training. But, after a few years, you may struggle to gain 0.5 kg/month. For example, if you weigh 70 kg at the start of your training programme, you could weigh as much as 76 kg after the first 3 months. This would then probably drop to about 1 kg/month, so after the first year you may weigh 85 kg – that's a gain of 15 kg. Don't expect to continue adding 6–12 kg a year every year, though. Your rate of weight gain will gradually drop off over the years as you approach your genetic potential. Also, the chances are you will have temporary and unavoidable breaks from your training programme – when you go on holiday or stop training due to illness, for example. Remember, your exact rate of weight gain will be influenced by your genetic potential. That's why two people can gain very different amounts of weight despite following the same training and eating programme. If you are putting on more than 3–4 kg/month, you are probably adding body fat, so you will need to cut down on your calorie intake.

SUMMARY OF KEY POINTS

- Muscles are made up of cylindrical fibres, which comprise bundles of filaments that hold the muscle proteins.
- The proportion of FT and ST muscle fibres influences your ability to develop strength, muscle mass and endurance.
- When a muscle contracts, the two contractile proteins, actin and myosin, slide across each other to shorten the muscle.
- Strength is the combined result of hypertrophy (increase in muscle size) and neuromuscular adaptation.
- Muscles increase in strength and mass when they are subjected to progressive overload.
- An increase in muscle size is due to an increase in muscle fibre size and density, not an increase in the number of fibres.
- The amount of lean weight you can gain depends on your genetic make-up, your natural body type, your mix of FT and ST muscle fibres, the arrangement of the motor units in your muscles and your hormonal balance, as well as the quality of your training and diet.
- Men can expect to gain 0.5–1 kg body weight/month; women can expect to gain 0.25–0.75 kg/month.
- Gains in the first year of training may be up to 20 per cent of starting body weight, then gradually slow down over the years.

PRINCIPLES AND METHODS OF STRENGTH TRAINING

3

Gaining a greater understanding of training principles and methods will help you target your training programme more effectively.

PROGRESSIVE TRAINING

Progressive resistance (or 'overload') training is a calculated method of progressively working your muscles harder and harder to induce gains in strength, mass or endurance. When you train with heavy weights, they adapt by getting stronger and stronger.

As you become stronger, fewer motor units (and therefore fewer muscle fibres) are needed to perform the same exercise (your muscles become more efficient at performing particular movements) so you have to subject your muscles to progressive amounts of overload. If you were to stick to the same workout – the same exercises, weights, sets, rep schemes and rep speeds – your muscles would stop adapting and growing, and you would only maintain your strength.

SETS AND REPS

The basic unit of resistance training is the repetition ('rep'). A repetition is one complete movement in the exercise, from the starting position to the point of maximum contraction and then back to the starting position. This ensures you complete what is called the full range of movement (ROM). On the bench press, for example, lowering the bar to your chest (the eccentric, or negative, part of the rep) and pushing it back up from your chest (the concentric, or positive, part of the rep) is 1 repetition.

These repetitions are grouped together in sets. If you perform 10 repetitions of the bench press before taking a rest, those 10 repetitions constitute a set.

One-rep max

One-rep max (1RM) is the heaviest weight that you can lift for 1 – and just 1 – repetition. In other words, you can do a maximum of 1 repetition only for a given weight. This can be calculated either directly (by performing your 1RM after a thorough warm-up) or indirectly by performing a 3RM (which is safer), then extrapolating this to what your 1RM should be. Alternatively, find a weight with which you can just perform 6 repetitions. This is equivalent to approximately 70–80 per cent of your 1RM.

TRAINING TO FAILURE

When training to failure, you perform repetitions until you can no longer lift the weight through the concentric (or positive) part of the movement using proper form. Each exercise has a 'sticking point' during the concentric phase – the part of the movement where gravity and unfavourable leverage make it hardest, and this is usually the part of the movement at which the point of muscular failure is reached. Training to the point of failure allows you to recruit the largest number of motor units, which in turn results in maximal muscle-fibre stimulation.

PYRAMID TRAINING

Pyramid training is a form of multiple-set training in which the weight is increased in each set and the number of repetitions reduced. This allows you to warm up a muscle group gradually, and prepare it over the course of a few sets to cope with heavier weights by the end of the sets – hence allowing the muscles to achieve greater overload, and allowing you to develop greater size and strength. A typical pyramid is shown in Figure 3.1. Select a weight that will enable you to reach near or complete failure at the end of each set.

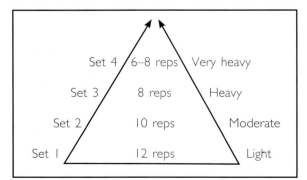

Figure 3.1 A typical pyramid pattern to increase muscle size

ECCENTRIC TRAINING ('NEGATIVES')

In eccentric training, a spotter assists you in lifting the bar (the concentric phase), and then you control the weight on the eccentric (lowering) phase. This technique allows you to use a heavier weight (110–160 per cent 1RM) so should be performed after a thorough warm-up and particularly at the end of a set after you have reached muscular failure. Focus on lowering the weight very slowly.

The principle behind this technique is that it produces greater muscle growth than conventional (concentric) training technique. During an eccentric contraction there is more mechanical load per motor unit. As a result, eccentric training can generate up to two-thirds more tension in the muscle than concentric training. Increased tension provides a greater stimulus to the muscle fibres which, in turn, means greater strength and growth.

As this is a very intense training method, limit eccentric training to one exercise per muscle group in any one workout, performing it at the end of only 1 or 2 sets. You will need to allow longer rest intervals between sets and, following hard eccentric training, you will experience greater muscle soreness because of the greater resulting muscle fibre damage. Recovery may take up to 10 days, so you should allow at least 10–14 days between muscle group workouts employing this technique. For example, if you perform eccentric training on the chest on Monday, do not use it for the chest again for two weeks.

FORCED, OR ASSISTED, REP TRAINING

With forced rep training you enlist the help of a spotter so that you can continue past the point of failure and therefore complete a couple of extra repetitions. The spotter should give just enough support to keep the weight moving through the sticking point.

You should only use this training technique for the last 1 or 2 reps of your heaviest sets, and should be able to complete at least 6 reps on your own in the correct form before the spotter assists you. If you cannot complete 6 reps, reduce the weight.

The advantage of forced rep training is that you can work past the point of muscular failure and thus increase the overload. For example, if you can normally complete 6 reps at 70 kg on the bench press, the forced rep training method may enable you to complete 8 reps, thus increasing the amount of stress that your pectorals receive. Whether this ultimately results in greater muscle hypertrophy, however, is a controversial issue. Like other advanced training methods, performing forced reps too frequently over an extended period may lead to overtraining and, ironically, a drop in performance. According to one study, performing forced reps after the point of failure does not lead to increased strength or power (Drinkwater *et al*, 2007).

Forced reps should only be used during intense training cycles and you should limit this method to once a week per muscle group.

DESCENDING (DROP) SETS

This method is particularly useful for reaching overload if you are training without a partner or spotter and cannot use eccentric or forced rep training.

With descending sets you complete as many repetitions in strict form as you can, then – without resting – you reduce the weight by 20–50 per cent and continue performing repetitions (usually 4–6) until you reach the point of failure again. Repeat this process if you wish.

Again, the objective is to stimulate as many motor units as possible. The first reps, performed with a heavy weight, stimulate the FT muscle fibres; subsequent reps performed with lighter weights stimulate mainly ST fibres. So this method allows you to train for strength, muscle size and endurance within the same set.

This method is safest for exercises with dumb-bells and machines since you need to be able to return the weight safely and quickly when your muscles have reached failure. Examples of suitable exercises include: leg extensions, leg curls, dumb-bell presses, flyes, lateral raises, dumbbell biceps curls, lat pull-downs, seated rows and triceps push-downs. For example, if you are performing a set of lateral raises with 10 kg dumbbells, complete as many reps as you can in strict form – say, eight. Return the dumbbells to the floor, pick up a pair of 7.5 kg dumbbells, and perform as many as you can until you reach failure – say, 5. Repeat with 5 kg dumbbells.

Since this method is very fatiguing, it should only be used for selected exercises and only for the last 1 or 2 sets, providing maximum stimulation to the muscle when it is fatigued. You will need to leave slightly longer rest intervals between descending sets (say 2–3 minutes) and reduce the total number of sets per muscle group. Again, use this method sparingly, once every 3 weeks.

SUPERSET TRAINING

This involves performing two or more exercises for a given body part in a row, and there are two methods, as described below.

Supersets for the same muscle groups

This method involves two or more exercises for the same muscle group – for example, dumbbell shoulder press followed by lateral raises and upright rows for the shoulders. The advantage is that the stress on the muscle is increased as the muscle can be worked from slightly different angles, thus involving more muscle fibres. It also increases the blood flow to the muscle due to the increased energy demand, providing greater stimulation for hypertrophy. However, this type of superset training should not be used for every body part or at every workout as it is very intense and may lead to overtraining.

Supersets for opposing muscle groups

This less intense method involves performing two exercises for opposing muscle groups – for example, biceps curls followed by triceps extensions, or leg extensions followed by leg curls. The advantage of this method is that the blood is kept within the same area of the body, thus encouraging a greater flow and bringing more fuel, oxygen and nutrients to the muscle. Since the rest period is eliminated, it is also a good way of reducing your workout time; this is particularly useful if you have only a limited period in which to train.

Unlike supersetting the same muscle group, this method does not significantly increase the muscle overload. However, it does increase the demands on your cardiovascular system since the rest periods are greatly reduced, and can therefore help to improve lactic acid tolerance, raise the anaerobic threshold and develop better stamina.

Following each superset you should take a 2–3 minute rest.

PRE-EXHAUSTION TRAINING

With pre-exhaustion training the larger muscle (prime mover) is partially exhausted by performing an isolation exercise prior to performing the compound exercise. For example, performing flyes before bench presses pre-exhausts the pectorals so that when you perform the bench presses, your pectorals will fatigue before, or at the same time as, the triceps and front deltoids. (You will probably need to reduce the weight you use for the bench presses.) There is no need to change the rest intervals between sets. The objective is to change the usual recruitment pattern of the muscle fibres involved and enable you to stimulate more muscle.

Like other advanced training methods, pre-exhaustion training should only be used for selected exercises and you should limit this method to once a week per muscle group.

Getting pumped

The 'pump' that you get during heavy training is not the same as muscle growth. This temporary increase in muscle size is largely the result of water accumulating inside the muscle fibres, making the muscle look larger. The majority of this water returns to the blood a few hours after training and so the pump disappears.

CORE TRAINING

Core training is based on the idea that by training the muscles surrounding the 'core' – torso, pelvis and spine – you can increase stability throughout your entire body. Training your 'core' also helps to build better balance and posture by aligning your body correctly, improve performance and prevent injury. When you work to strengthen and stabilise your core, you strengthen your body's power base.

Core stability

Core stability refers to the long-term training of the deep postural muscles (stabilisers) that support the spine. One way of training these muscles is to work from an unstable base such as an exercise ball or BOSU ball.

There are many exercises that challenge core stability. Pilates is one of the best-known stability programmes, others involve exercising from an unstable base such as a wobble board or exercise ball. This places a higher demand on the deep muscles in the core – or trunk – as well as on your motor control system because you constantly have to stabilise yourself as the ball or board rolls around. It also changes the way your neuromuscular system coordinates movement as you're using your legs to hold you up, and your abdominals and back to keep your whole body stable. Traditional exercises have little effect on core stability as they do not work the trunk stabilisers – the transverse abdominis (TVA) and the lumbar multifidus – but doing exercises on a ball or wobble board challenges stability on many planes of movement, so works these muscles more effectively.

The first step in core training is to find your neutral posture, where your joints are aligned correctly to each other. To locate this, follow the steps outlined below.

- Stand with your feet hip-width apart, knees relaxed.
- Let your shoulders drop down and away from your ears.
- Lengthen your spine and neck – imagine a string, attached to the top of your head, pulling you up to the ceiling.
- Contract your abdominal muscles, drawing the navel in towards your spine.
- Adjust the tilt of your pelvis so that it is in a neutral position. You should be able to draw a line vertically from your shoulders to your hips to your feet.

Once you have mastered maintaining your neutral posture, you will be training your core muscles during any activity. Try to integrate core training into your weights workouts. Maintain tension in your abdominals and keep your spine in neutral alignment at all times.

Seated exercises, such as shoulder presses or biceps curls, can be performed on an exercise ball. Hold in your abdominals and keep your back in the neutral posture – your shoulders and hips should form a straight line. Try using an exercise ball instead of a bench for doing lying dumbbell presses and flyes. Not only will you target your chest but you'll also be working your core muscles to maintain balance and stability on the ball. You will need to use lighter weights than usual.

TRAINING WITH AN EXERCISE BALL

Exercise (stability) balls will add intensity and interest to your usual programme – using a ball instead of a bench immediately adds depth to moves such as dumbbell presses, and engages more muscle groups. They are widely used by athletes, weight trainers, coaches and personal trainers for developing balance and core strength. Because the ball is an unstable surface, you work on those small, vital stability muscles of the legs and torso even while you're doing other things like strengthening the back in back extensions, or the chest in push-ups. You can use the ball as a weight bench, a place to sit and a support for so many exercises, so you can move through exercises quickly without needing a lot of extra equipment. You can also use it for stretching, yoga, Pilates and even sitting at your desk or in front of the TV.

Exercises performed on an exercise ball will improve your core strength and posture. Being round, the ball wants to roll away so you have to use your postural muscles to maintain balance. When you lie on the ball, your legs and abs immediately contract to keep you from falling off. Add an exercise to that (like a chest press or a crunch), and you increase the intensity of the movement.

However, when performing exercises with weights on the ball, such as a chest press or shoulder press, you'll find that you won't be able to use quite as much weight compared with performing the exercise on a stable surface. This isn't disadvantageous: you're still generating the same force in the working muscles and increasing joint stability, which will help prevent injury.

It can also be used for increasing the range of movement in abdominal and lower back exercises. This is advantageous because it allows you to work a greater amount of muscle. For example, doing an abdominal crunch on the ball allows the abdominals to work through a greater range compared with doing the same exercise on the floor. At the same time, other muscles must work to stabilise you on the ball. So, not only are you strengthening your abdominals and postural muscles but you are also improving your balance.

Using an exercise ball can help with back problems in sedentary people. Studies have found that exercise ball training does improve spinal stability, noting that this kind of training would be beneficial to individuals who spend a good deal of time sitting, or for those who are prone to back pain but have been cleared to exercise (Carter *et al*, 2006; Sekendiz *et al*, 2011; Willardson, 2007).

Before you buy a ball, make sure it's the right size for your height. To test it, sit on the ball and make sure your hips are level with or just slightly higher than the knees:

Ball diameter	Your height
55 cm	1.5m–1.65m (4'11"–5'4")
65 cm	1.65m–1.8m (5'5"–5'11")
75 cm	1.8m–2m (6'0"–6'7")

- **Resistance training**. Use the exercise ball as a weight bench to add difficulty to the movements and incorporate the muscles of your legs, butt and abs.
- **Abdominal training**. Doing crunches, twists and other exercises on the ball adds difficulty to the movement by recruiting more muscles.
- **Sitting around**. Just sitting on an exercise ball can be a challenge and it's a great way to improve your posture when sitting in front of a computer or watching television.
- **Flexibility, yoga and Pilates exercises**. The ball is great for stretching and relaxing.

TRAINING WITH A BOSU BALL/ BALANCE TRAINER

The BOSU ('both sides up') ball is like an exercise ball that's been cut in half with a platform on the bottom. The squishy dome side on top and flat platform on the bottom allow you to use the ball in many ways, which will add variety to your workouts. You can use it dome-side-up for cardio, lower body strength, or core moves. Or, you can turn it over and use the platform side for upper body exercises, like push-ups, or more core moves, like planks.

Using the BOSU ball can help to improve balance because you're constantly engaging the small stabiliser muscles in the upper and lower body to keep you in place. When you stand on, or perform exercises with, a BOSU ball, all of your muscles are forced to contract to keep your joints in proper position as you try to maintain your centre of gravity over an unstable surface. It also helps improve kinesthetic awareness (your sense of how the body is positioned at any given moment) and proprioception (how your body responds to external forces to keep your joints in the right position).

- **Cardio** Use the BOSU ball for short bursts of cardio such as hops, jumps, step-ups, leaps and lunges.
- **Strength training** Add a new challenge to your squats, lunges, deadlifts and push-ups. You can even use the BOSU ball as a weight bench to add a balance challenge during traditional weight work.
- **Flexibility** Stand or kneel on the dome while doing traditional stretches to add more range of motion.
- **Sports conditioning** Use it to perform sports drills, like jumping or plyometric moves, to increase performance and agility.
- **Core training** Use it for abdominal and lower back exercises to target the core muscles.

TRAINING WITH RESISTANCE BANDS

Resistance bands can also provide a good strength workout, and be just as challenging as machines or dumbbells. You can perform the same exercises as you do with free weights – the difference lies in positioning the band. For example, you can stand on the band and grip the handles for biceps curls or overhead presses. You can attach it to a door and do lat pull-downs or triceps push-downs. You can wrap the band around a pole for chest exercises or shoulder rotations. The possibilities are endless. If you use good form and the right level of tension, your muscles won't know the difference between weights or bands. Plus, bands offer more variety because you can create the resistance from all directions – the side, overhead, below, etc.

When you use free weights, gravity decides where the weight comes from, so you get more resistance during one part of the movement (such as the upswing of a biceps curl) than the other (the downswing). With bands, the tension is constant, which makes it feel harder.

Other benefits include:

- They are portable. You can easily pack them in your bag for travel and do exercises away from the gym.
- They increase coordination. Because there's tension throughout the exercises, you have to stabilise your body. This helps with coordination and balance, and it also helps you to involve more muscle groups.
- They add variety. With weights, there is a limited number of exercises. But the resistance band allows you to change your positioning in multiple ways. This changes how an exercise feels.

- They are cheap.
- They're great for all fitness levels. Depending on how you use them, bands can be great for beginners as well as more advanced exercisers. You can use them for basic moves or to add intensity to traditional moves.

PERIODISATION

Periodisation refers to the planned manipulation of training volume and intensity throughout a series of specific training phases or cycles. It is an application of the principles of progressive training (you vary your repetitions, sets, weight and intensity during each cycle) and is a method used to make continual improvements in performance throughout the year, thus avoiding reaching plateaux. If you follow the same workout for any length of time, the body soon adapts to the constant load and your gains diminish. However, by structuring your long-term training goals in a number of training cycles, you will be able to make gains in strength, mass and definition all year round, and will also avoid overtraining and injury.

Proof that periodisation works better than sticking to the same routine week after week comes from a review of studies at Appalachian State University in Boone, North Carolina, and the USA Weightlifting Development Center in Shreveport, Louisiana (Stone *et al*, 1999). The experienced weight trainers who followed a periodised programme made significant improvements in strength (as measured by their 1RM for the squat), whereas those who followed a standard programme did not show any improvement.

A periodisation programme is divided into a number of distinct cycles. The longest cycle is called a macrocycle and usually spans a period of 1 year, although shorter macrocycles can be used – for example, two macrocycles per year are used in a double-periodisation programme. This would suit those who cannot commit themselves to a year-round programme or those who want greater variety in their training.

The year is then broken down into 2–6 shorter training cycles (mesocycles), each spanning several weeks. Each mesocycle emphasises a particular training goal (e.g. muscle size or muscular endurance) and involves a gradual increase in training intensity. The aim is to peak at the end of your mesocycle. For strength trainers, this may be gauged by the amount of weight that can be lifted.

Each mesocycle is then followed by a short period (1–2 weeks) of relative rest, which is important to allow your body to recover and recuperate before beginning the next mesocycle. Provided this rest phase lasts no longer than 4 weeks, you will not experience a detraining effect. During this time, you should do only very light training, or a different activity such as golf or recreational swimming, that does not tax your energy systems or central nervous system in the same way.

Each mesocycle is then divided into week-long microcycles, around which you plan your day-to-day workouts.

There are many variations on periodisation programmes, dependent on your goals, training experience and lifestyle. The examples given on the following pages may be used as a basis for designing your own programme. You may commence training at any time during the year – simply change the month headings. The important point is to follow the mesocycles in the given order, and to gradually increase your training intensity within each mesocycle.

PERIODISATION PROGRAMME 1: MUSCULAR ENDURANCE

Aims
1. Improve muscular endurance
2. Improve muscle tone

This periodisation programme emphasises muscular endurance and comprises four mesocycles of circuit training, each progressively increasing in intensity. Shortening the rest intervals from 30 seconds to 20 seconds, adding more circuits to your allocated workout time, and changing the reps and weight achieve this. If you are training for a particular sport, include exercises that work the main muscle groups involved in that sport and that mimic the movements used (e.g. lat pull-down if you are a swimmer). You can also concentrate on particular goals:

- muscular strength and endurance – use slightly heavier weights for 12–15 reps, with slightly longer rest intervals between exercises
- cardiovascular fitness/fat loss – use lighter weights for up to 20 reps, with a cardiovascular exercise such as the stationary bike or jogging between stations.

Table 3.1	Periodisation programme 1 – to improve muscular endurance (beginners)

Macrocycle

Jan.	Feb.	Mar.	Apr.	May	June	July	Aug.	Sept.	Oct.	Nov.	Dec.
	Mesocycle 1			Mesocycle 2			Mesocycle 3			Mesocycle 4	
	12 weeks ME	1 week R	12 weeks ME		1 week R	12 weeks ME		1 week R	12 weeks ME		1 week R

Progression

Reduce rest interval between sets from 30 to 15 seconds
Increase repetitions from 15 to a maximum of 20
Increase number of circuits performed in 45 minutes
Use slightly heavier weights if you can exceed 20 reps

Key:
ME = muscle endurance training (see pp. 210–216)
R = rest/low-intensity activity

PERIODISATION PROGRAMME 2: MUSCLE SIZE (BEGINNERS)

Aims
1. Increase muscle size
2. Increase strength

This cycle includes a 12-week muscular endurance mesocycle to build a good base of conditioning and prepare the muscles for the next mesocycles. The exact length of the muscle size mesocycles will depend on your level of conditioning and any holiday commitments. For example, you may need to shorten mesocycle 1 to avoid overtraining. As you become adapted to training, however, you should be able to sustain the full training cycles. Increase the intensity gradually by using progressively heavier weights.

Table 3.2	Periodisation programme 2 – to improve muscle size (beginners)

Macrocycle

Jan.	Feb.	Mar.	Apr.	May	June	July	Aug.	Sept.	Oct.	Nov.	Dec.

| Mesocycle 1 | | | | Mesocycle 2 | | | | Mesocycle 3 | | Mesocycle 4 | |

| 12 weeks ME | 1 week R | 10 weeks ME | 3 weeks R | 10 weeks ME | 3 weeks R | 4 weeks MS | 2 weeks MS | 4 weeks MS | 2 weeks AMS | 1 week R |

Progression
Gradually increase weight used in each mesocycle

Key:
ME = muscle endurance training (see pp. 210–216)
MS = muscle size training (see pp. 217–222)
AMS = advanced muscle size training (see pp. 224–225 – descending (drop) set workout)
R = rest/low-intensity activity

PERIODISATION PROGRAMME 3: MUSCLE SIZE (INTERMEDIATE AND ADVANCED)

Aims
1. Increase muscle size
2. Increase strength

This plan is suitable for weight trainers with at least 1–2 years' experience. Following a 6-week mesocycle, building muscle endurance and strength, this periodisation programme emphasises muscle hypertrophy. Muscle size cycles dominate, interspersed with short periods that incorporate advanced training methods – descending (drop) sets, supersets and pre-exhaustion – and maximum strength training methods. The objective is to avoid training plateaux and produce long-term muscle size gains.

Table 3.3	Periodisation programme 3 – to improve muscle size (intermediate and advanced)

Macrocycle

Jan.	Feb.	Mar.	Apr.	May	June	July	Aug.	Sept.	Oct.	Nov.	Dec.

Mesocycle 1 | | | **Mesocycle 2** | | | | **Mesocycle 3** | | | **Mesocycle 4**

6 weeks ME | 1 week R | 6 weeks MS | 1 week R | 6 weeks MS | 1 week R | 2 weeks AMS | 4 weeks MS | 1 week R | 2 weeks AMS | 4 weeks MS | 1 week R | 4 weeks MS | 4 weeks MS | 4 weeks MXS | 1 week R

Progression
Gradually increase amount of weight used

Key:
ME = muscle endurance training (see pp. 210–216)
MS = muscle size training (see pp. 217–222)
AMS = advanced muscle size training (see pp. 223–229 – any of the 3 workouts)
MXS = maximum strength training (see pp. 230–231)
R = rest/low-intensity activity

PERIODISATION PROGRAMME 4: MAXIMUM STRENGTH (ADVANCED)

Aims
1. Increase maximum strength
2. Promote long-term hypertrophy

This periodisation programme is suitable for advanced weight trainers who want to develop stronger muscles and long-term hypertrophy. Following a 6-week conditioning mesocycle to prepare the body for the forthcoming intense training, the programme incorporates both maximum strength training methods and advanced muscle size training methods. Muscle strength training cycles dominate and are interspersed with advanced training method cycles and maximum strength training.

Table 3.4	Periodisation programme 4 – to increase maximum strength (advanced)

Macrocycle											
Jan.	Feb.	Mar.	Apr.	May	June	July	Aug.	Sept.	Oct.	Nov.	Dec.
Mesocycle 1		Mesocycle 2			Mesocycle 3			Mesocycle 4		Mesocycle 5	
6 weeks ME	1 week R	6 weeks MS	6 weeks MXS	1 week R	6 weeks MXS	3 weeks MS	2 weeks R	3 weeks MXS	3 weeks MS	3 weeks AMS	1 week R	4 weeks MXS	2 weeks AMS	3 weeks MXS	2 weeks R

Progression
Gradually increase amount of weight used

Key:
ME = muscle endurance training (see pp. 210–216)
MS = muscle size training (see pp. 217–222)
AMS = advanced muscle size training (see pp. 223–229 – any of the 3 workouts)
MXS = maximum strength training (see pp. 230–231)
R = rest/low-intensity activity

SUMMARY OF KEY POINTS

- Set training and pyramid training form the core of any training programme for strength, power or size.
- Advanced training methods – such as eccentric training, forced rep training, descending sets, supersets and pre-exhaustion – allow you to train with greater intensity and experience continued gains.
- Core training can be integrated into weights workouts to improve balance, posture and performance, prevent injury and strengthen the lower back.

PROGRAMME DESIGN

Understanding the components of a training programme will help you to work out more effectively and achieve your goals. There are several key variables, which you can manipulate to meet your goals (Bompa & Cornacchia, 1998; Baechle & Earle, 2000; Fleck & Kraemer, 1997).

SELECTION OF EXERCISES

The exercises you select for your programme should result in equal stimulation of each muscle group, and ensure that no muscle group is left out.

Keep your muscles growing by having a greater repertoire of exercises from which to choose. You can do this by frequently changing the exercises you perform for each muscle group and by using variations of standard exercises in different body positions to emphasise different parts of the muscle group.

COMPOUND VS ISOLATION EXERCISES

Compound, or multi-joint, exercises cause greatest stimulation of the muscle fibres and should form the basis of strength- and mass-building programmes. They involve one or more large muscle groups (i.e. the chest, legs, shoulders, back, hips) and work across two or more major joints. For example, the bench press is a compound exercise that is used primarily to target the pectoral muscles but also involves the triceps and front deltoids. Therefore, the exercise stimulates three muscle groups. It is a multi-joint exercise because the movement involves both arm flexion (the shoulder joint) and extension of the forearm (the elbow joint).

Isolation, or single-joint, exercises involve smaller muscle groups (i.e. biceps, triceps, brachioradialis, erector spinae) and only one main joint. For example, the dumbbell flye is an isolation exercise that is used primarily to target the pectorals. The elbows are kept at a fixed angle throughout the ROM and so no other muscle groups are worked. It is a single-joint exercise as it only works around the shoulder joint.

Isolation exercises are often included in beginner programmes because they are easier to learn and execute using good form. Once you have mastered the basic movement patterns, plan your programme around compound exercises that stimulate a greater number of muscle fibres.

THE PRINCIPLE OF SPECIFICITY

The principle of exercise specificity means that your body will adapt to the specific demands imposed on them. In other words, if you do a particular movement you will get better at that movement. If you do a partial range of motion, you will get stronger in that range of motion only. Similarly, if you use light weights for a high number of reps you will increase your muscular endurance. If you use medium or heavy weights then you will gain strength and muscle mass.

ORDER OF EXERCISES

The order in which you perform your exercises will affect the energy and effort you are able to put into the next exercise. For example, performing two consecutive exercises that both stimulate the same muscle group reduces the effort you can put into the second one. The order can be changed according to the aspect of strength you wish to develop, and there are four methods, as outlined below.

1. LARGEST TO SMALLEST

The most usual way of ordering exercises is to work from the largest muscle groups to the smallest. Therefore, compound exercises that stimulate the largest muscle groups are performed first in your workout, followed by the isolation exercises. This is because the compound exercises require the most effort and concentration and are very difficult to perform correctly and safely if your muscles are fatigued. For example, in a leg workout you would perform compound exercises such as squats and leg presses before isolation exercises such as leg extensions and leg curls.

Advanced trainers sometimes reverse this order to break through a training plateau. This is called pre-exhaustion and involves deliberately fatiguing a large muscle group by performing isolation exercises before the compound exercise (see p. 36).

2. ALTERNATING UPPER- AND LOWER-BODY CIRCUIT

Alternating upper- and lower-body exercises is particularly suitable for beginners who might find performing several exercises for one area in one go too demanding. This method allows each muscle group to recover more fully between exercises, and is also good for people with limited training time available because it minimises rest intervals – you can perform an upper-body exercise straight after a lower-body exercise without resting. Because rest periods are minimised, you also get a greater cardiovascular effect compared with more conventional strength training programmes. On the downside, this method generally results in less stimulation of each muscle group, and can result in slower strength and mass gains. Therefore, it would be less suitable for advanced weight trainers.

3. ALTERNATING 'PUSH' AND 'PULL' EXERCISES

Alternating pushing exercises (e.g. bench press) and pulling exercises (e.g. seated row) is also suitable for beginners, those resuming strength training and those with limited training time available. As with alternating upper- and lower-body exercises, this method is a very good way of reducing your rest periods because, while you are performing a pulling exercise (the seated row), the opposing muscle group used in the pushing exercise (the bench press) is recovering. You will not need to rest, yet you can still use maximum effort for each set. If you were to arrange several pushing exercises together (e.g. bench press, shoulder press, triceps extensions), you might have to reduce the amount of weight or number of repetitions used because the triceps (a muscle used in all three exercises) will become fatigued.

4. SUPERSETS

This training method involves two or more sets of different exercises performed consecutively with no rest period between. As it is very demanding, supersets are best suited to advanced weight trainers (see pp. 226, 227).

SETS AND REPS

The number of sets and reps you perform depends on your goals, training experience, the number of muscle groups trained per session, and the size of the muscle group being trained.

Table 4.1 gives guidelines for the number of sets and repetitions, weight and rest intervals commonly prescribed for strength, power, hypertrophy and muscular endurance training programmes.

MAXIMUM STRENGTH

Maximum strength is developed using heavy weights and low-repetition sets. The consensus guideline is to perform 2–6 sets of 6 or fewer repetitions for the compound exercises (Bompa & Cornacchia, 1998; Fleck & Kraemer, 1997; Tan, 1999). Only 1–3 sets are necessary for isolation exercises (Hass *et al*, 2000). Clearly you should select a weight that causes you to use maximum effort for that set – that is, reach the point of failure on the last repetition (between 85 and 100 per cent 1RM). Your rest intervals between sets should be 3–4 minutes to allow sufficient recovery. Maximum strength workouts are centred on the compound exercises such as squats, bench presses and shoulder presses.

POWER

Performing an exercise very quickly or explosively develops power. It can be developed with plyometrics and speed drills, as well as weightlifting exercises. For example, squat jumps and alternate leg bounding (plyometrics), 40 m dashes, shuttle runs (speed drills), power cleans, power pulls or any compound resistance training exercises (e.g.

Table 4.1	Sets, repetitions, weight and rest interval guidelines for different training goals				
Training goal	Number of sets per exercise	Number of repetitions	Weight (% 1RM)	Rest interval	Training tempo*
Maximum strength	2–6	< 6	Heavy (> 85)	2–5 min	1:2
Power	3–5	1–5	Heavy (75–85)	2–5 min	Explosive:1
Muscle size	3–6	6–12	67–85	30–90 s	2:3
Muscular endurance	2–3	> 12	Low (< 67)	< 30 s	2:3

*The training tempo is the number of counts for the concentric (lifting) action, followed by the number of counts for the eccentric (lowering) action, e.g. 2:3 is 2 counts concentric, 3 counts eccentric.

leg press, squat) performed explosively would all be suitable methods of developing neuromuscular activity and power (see page 234 – power workout). Power exercises would be suitable for intermediate and advanced weight trainers, Olympic lifters, and athletes who use power movements in their particular sport. For example, basketball, football, sprinting and most field athletic events (such as the high jump and long jump) involve explosive activities, so power training would benefit your performance.

However, only experienced lifters and athletes should use this type of training as it could be dangerous if attempted using imperfect technique. It is important that the weight is kept under good control even when it is moved rapidly. The consensus guideline is 3–5 sets of 1–5 repetitions (Bompa & Cornacchia, 1998; Baechle & Groves, 1998), using moderate (75–85 per cent 1RM), rather than maximal, weights. Slightly lighter weights allow you to perform the exercise with maximum speed and therefore generate the greatest power output: output almost doubles when reducing the weight from 100 per cent 1RM to 90 per cent 1RM (Garhammer & McLaughlin, 1980).

MUSCLE SIZE

Training for muscle size (hypertrophy) requires a higher training volume compared with pure strength and power training – in other words, more repetitions, sets and a greater cumulative amount of weight lifted per workout. The consensus guideline is a moderate number of repetitions (6–12) and 3–6 sets per exercise performed with a moderate to heavy weight (67–85 per cent 1RM) and short to moderate rest intervals (30–90 seconds) (Bompa & Cornacchia, 1998; Fleck & Kraemer, 1997; Hedrick, 1995).

You can expect parallel increases in both muscle size and strength with this type of training programme. For overall size development, your programme should be based around compound exercises that stimulate the large muscle groups (e.g. squats, bench presses, shoulder presses, lat pull-downs). More advanced weight trainers and bodybuilders use 2–4 exercises per muscle group, including at least one or two compound exercises. They use a split training system (see below), allowing them to train with high intensity.

MUSCULAR ENDURANCE

Muscular endurance is the ability of a muscle or muscle group to sustain sub-maximal force over a period of time. This type of training increases the aerobic capacity of the muscles rather than muscle size and strength, and is developed by using a higher number of repetitions (12 or more) per set and minimal rest intervals between sets – typically less than 30 seconds (Bompa & Cornacchia, 1998; Fleck & Kraemer, 1997). The weights lifted are lighter and fewer sets are performed per muscle group, usually 2 or 3. Therefore, the intensity is very low and the overall volume high.

This type of workout is suitable for beginners but also for advanced weight trainers wishing to improve this aspect of their fitness. Most circuit resistance training programmes, which alternate upper-and lower-body exercises or opposing muscle groups and limit rest intervals to 30 seconds or less, would promote muscular endurance.

FULL-BODY ROUTINE VS SPLIT WORKOUTS

If you plan to train all major muscle groups in your workout (a full-body routine), you should perform 1 or 2 sets of each exercise and only 1

How fast should you lift?

Perhaps the most important principle for stimulating muscle growth is the time that the muscle is under tension – i.e. the time your muscles are actually working. For example, if you blast a set of 10 repetitions as fast as possible, your total time under tension will be just a few seconds. This is not sufficient to cause your muscles to grow, regardless of the amount of weight you lift. Typically, the time under tension should be 30–70 seconds. Anything more or less would be counterproductive and result in very little gain.

The way to achieve the correct set duration is to adjust your training tempo. For example, if you are working in relatively low-rep ranges (say, 6–8), you will have to adjust your training tempo – particularly on the eccentric (lowering) part of the movement – in order for that set's time under tension to reach at least 30 seconds. If you are working in a higher-rep range (say, 10–12), the training tempo should be a little quicker so that you won't exceed the 30–70 seconds' time under tension range.

When does detraining begin?

It is a myth that loss of strength and muscle mass begins within 72 hours of a workout. Since it may take several days for compensation to occur following a heavy workout, it would not be possible for decompensation to begin in such a short time. For this reason, many experienced weight trainers train only major muscle groups once a week. Indeed, many weight trainers have experienced dramatic increases in growth using this method.

TRAINING INTENSITY

Training intensity serves as the major stimulus for muscle growth. By increasing your training intensity, you provide a bigger stimulus for muscle growth. You can increase the intensity by increasing the amount of weight, number of sets or repetitions, and the number of exercises, or reducing rest intervals between sets. The exact combination you choose depends on your goals, strength, power, size or muscular endurance.

REST PERIODS BETWEEN WORKOUTS

Rest between workouts is as important as the training itself. This is when replenishment, recovery, adaptation and growth take place. Let's take a look at what happens.

During and immediately after a workout your body is in a catabolic state (i.e. breaking down proteins) and levels of stress hormones such as cortisol are high. As you start to recover from your workout, levels of muscle-promoting hormones such as testosterone gradually rise, the damaged

or 2 exercises per muscle group, making a total of 15–20 sets.

As you progress to a split routine, dividing your whole-body workout into 2 or 3 separate workouts, you will be able to perform more sets per muscle group. The larger muscle groups (legs, back, chest, shoulders) generally require more sets (e.g. 6–12) than the smaller muscle groups (biceps, triceps), which require fewer sets (e.g. 3–8) for the advanced weight trainer to achieve sufficient stimulation.

muscle proteins are replaced with new muscle proteins, and glycogen stores are also restored. Clearly, these processes take time. It is only after completion of the recovery process that the muscles can grow and strengthen. If you attempt to train your muscles before the process is complete then you will experience only minimal growth or none at all. In other words, training before you have recovered fully is counterproductive.

The rest period you need to leave between workouts depends on the intensity and duration of your workout, your training experience and your diet.

TRAINING INTENSITY AND DURATION

The more intense your workout, the longer the recovery time required before your next training session. There is no easy or accurate way of predicting your recovery time between workouts. In the laboratory, scientists can measure the blood levels of muscle metabolites such as 3-methyl histidine and creatine phosphokinase, but this is clearly not a practical solution for everyday training. Instead, a certain amount of guesswork is required as you have to judge the 'feel' of your muscles. When your muscles have regained their pre-workout capacity – measured by testing your strength – you have probably recovered. Obviously, if your muscles still feel sore, stiff or weak, then they have not recovered. If you find yourself stronger and able to work out harder, then you know your muscles have recovered fully.

In general, upper-body muscles can recover more quickly from heavy workouts than lower-body muscles. Also, it takes longer to recover from compound exercises than isolation exercises.

TRAINING EXPERIENCE

The American College of Sports Medicine (ACSM) recommends that beginners train 2 or 3 times a week on non-consecutive days. As you become more experienced and better conditioned, you can increase your workout frequency to 4 or more times a week.

As a general guideline, beginners should leave a minimum of 1 day and a maximum of 3 days' recovery between workouts. Experienced weight trainers will need to leave 3–7 days between training the same muscle group due to the greater workout intensity. However, you can train 4 or more times a week by using a split routine – that is, dividing your major muscle groups into 2 or more separate workouts (see Part 4). That way, you can still allow a minimum of 3 days' rest between training each muscle group.

YOUR DIET

During recovery, your muscle glycogen stores are replenished and muscle tissue repaired. The time it takes to replenish muscle glycogen depends on the severity of depletion, and the amount and timing of carbohydrate intake in your diet. On average, this takes between 24 hours and 3 days. You also need to ensure you consume enough protein to provide the raw material for new muscle growth. An inadequate intake will result in slower repair and growth, and so your strength gains will be compromised. On the other hand, an excessive intake will not further enhance muscle growth or strength.

PROPER TRAINING TECHNIQUE

Training with proper form is crucial to avoid injury and maximise results. Your muscles don't know how much weight is on the bar but they do respond to the magnitude of tension developed during each movement. High levels of tension are achieved with proper form and relatively heavy weights. Many weight trainers get into the habit of using poor training form in order to lift more weight or squeeze out a couple of extra repetitions, but that does not produce better results. If you are unsure of an exercise, get assistance from an instructor or personal trainer who will be able to reinforce good technique. Pay close attention to the descriptions for each exercise in Part Three of this book and the following technique tips:

1. Always warm up properly before starting your workout. Never train a cold muscle as this increases injury risk.
2. Select a weight that will allow you to complete the desired number of repetitions safely. Do not be tempted to lift heavier weights before you have developed sufficient strength in your muscles, tendons and ligaments.
3. The general rule of thumb is to breathe out on the concentric (or positive) part of the movement (when you lift the weight) and breathe in on the eccentric (or negative) part of the movement (lowering the weight). Never hold your breath.
4. Perform each repetition using the complete ROM, taking the muscle from its fully extended position to its fully contracted position. Partial repetitions will develop strength only in that portion of the movement, and produce only slow overall gains. Also avoid cheating movements as these will reduce the training stimulus and increase injury risk.
5. Maintain full control of the weight throughout the movement. Swinging a weight too fast means momentum takes over to bear the load rather than the target muscles, putting your joints at risk of injury.
6. Focus on both the concentric and eccentric phases of each movement. Resist the weight as you bring it slowly to the starting position.
7. To find the correct training tempo, count to 2 as you lift the weight, and count to 3 as you lower it. Hold the fully contracted position for a count of 1 (but do not relax) before returning the weight to the starting position.
8. Visualising your target muscle contracting and relaxing will not only help you perform the exercise with good technique but will also help you do more repetitions. For example, as you press the bar up for a bench press, visualise your chest muscles contracting and getting stronger. This strategy reinforces the powerful mind–body link, which gives you more control over your body and, ultimately, greater physical gains.
9. Ideally, stretch the target muscles between sets, holding each stretch for a minimum of eight seconds.
10. Perform longer (developmental) stretches immediately after the workout. Each stretch should be held for 30–60 seconds.

TROUBLESHOOTING

Many trainers fail to make significant progress despite many months or years of training. Initial gains in muscular endurance and muscle tone are relatively rapid in beginners but gains in muscle size and strength can be painstakingly slow after the first 6 months. To make improvements on a regular basis, you need to look carefully at every aspect of your training programme.

CHOOSING THE WRONG EXERCISES

The selection of exercises in your programme depends on your specific goals and your training experience. For example, if your goal is to increase muscle size, you have to prioritise maximal-stimulation or compound exercises (e.g. squats, bench presses, barbell rows, shoulder presses) in your programme. These stimulate the largest muscles and the greatest proportion of fibres in those muscles. Isolation exercises (e.g. triceps kickbacks, biceps curls), which work smaller muscle groups or a smaller proportion of the muscle fibres in that muscle group, should be kept to a minimum and performed last in your workout.

DOING TOO MANY REPETITIONS

If you can do more than about 12 repetitions, it means that you are using too light a weight to stimulate growth in the FT muscle fibres. Doing more than 12 repetitions will improve muscular endurance but produce only small improvements in strength and size. Therefore, if it is muscle growth you want, select a weight that will allow you to perform 6–12 repetitions. Using a heavier weight that allows you to perform no more than 6 repetitions will improve your maximum strength. This method will not produce maximum size but can be useful for overcoming training plateaux within a hypertrophy programme.

DOING TOO MANY SETS

Research has established that less is best when it comes to building size and mass. The exact number of sets required to achieve maximal stimulation of the muscle fibres is debatable. The general recommendation for muscle size is 8–12 sets for larger muscle groups and 3–8 sets for smaller muscle groups, but the most important goal is to achieve overload. Whether you achieve this after 1 set or 12 is less important.

Advocates of single-set training claim overload can be achieved by performing a strict set of 6–10 repetitions with a heavy weight to failure, following a few warm-up sets. Once overload has been achieved, there is no benefit in performing further sets. Doing too many sets also leads to glycogen depletion and increased protein (muscle) breakdown, creating a net catabolic (breakdown) state – just the opposite of your goal! If you can perform more sets than the recommended range, this means you have failed to train hard enough to reach overload and stimulate growth.

NOT ENOUGH REST

If you don't give your body enough rest between workouts, you will not experience gains in mass or strength. One of the biggest mistakes made by beginners in their desire to make rapid gains is training too frequently. It is tempting to think that the more often you train, the faster you will gain mass, but in fact the opposite is true. Growth can only take place after compensation and full recovery. In other words, training before you have fully recovered can lead to a net protein (muscle) breakdown and, over time, can lead to overtraining. As a general guideline, beginners should leave 1–3 days' recovery between workouts, while experienced weight trainers should leave 3–7 days between training the same muscle group due to the greater workout intensity.

LACK OF PROGRESSION

Many weight trainers become disheartened when strength gains slow down or plateau despite maintaining a consistent workout programme. Indeed, it is easy to get stuck in a rut if you use the same weights, same exercises and same number of sets and reps. The muscles can soon adapt to a routine programme if the stimulus remains the same. In order to continue making strength and mass gains, your training programme must be progressive. That is, you must continue to increase the amount of stimulus applied. This may be achieved in one of the following ways:

- change the number of reps – either increase them up to a maximum of 12 (for developing muscle size), or decrease them to 3–6, using a heavier weight (for developing maximum strength)
- increase the number of sets – up to a maximum of 12 for major muscle groups and eight for smaller muscle groups
- change the type of exercises you perform and vary your workout – e.g. if you always perform lat pull-downs, seated rows and close-grip chins for your back, change to wide-grip chins, one arm dumbbell rows and pull-overs
- use different variations of exercises – e.g. different grip distances or foot positions (see the wide range of variations outlined in Part 3)
- change the order of your exercises – e.g. instead of always working from the largest to the smallest muscle groups, use the pre-exhaustion method for one workout, or try new sequences such as alternating pushing and pulling exercises, or using supersets either for the same muscle group or for opposing muscle groups
- change the training tempo – e.g. take shorter rest periods between sets
- use advanced training methods – e.g. eccentric training, forced or assisted reps, descending sets or supersets

- change the training split – e.g. train your shoulders and back together instead of your shoulders and arms.

PARTIAL RANGE OF MOVEMENT

If you use an incomplete ROM, the muscle fibres receive only partial stimulation. You may be able to use a heavier weight doing partial repetitions but the overall stimulus applied will be greatly reduced. This is a very common fault made by weight trainers keen to increase the weight lifted – but it is at the expense of correct form. Research has proved that taking a movement to the end of its natural range produces a more powerful anabolic stimulus than exercising over an incomplete ROM. It also produces better muscle shape, and prevents muscle shortening and reduced flexibility. You will therefore achieve considerably greater gains by performing each repetition through its complete ROM, even if it means using a lighter weight to do so.

POOR TECHNIQUE

Many weight trainers sacrifice technique in an attempt to lift heavier weights. Not only does this increase the risk of injury but it limits gains in strength and mass. 'Cheating' movements – such as arching the back and bouncing the bar off the chest when performing a bench press, bending forwards excessively when squatting or swinging backwards when doing barbell curls – reduce the work done by the prime mover muscles and put the back at risk of injury. Correct technique is therefore vital in order to make continued gains in strength and mass.

AVOIDANCE OF GOAL-SETTING

It is essential to set goals if you want to achieve results (see p. 50). First, be clear about exactly what you want to achieve, setting specific goals (e.g. 'I want to gain 5 kg of muscle') that are measurable and realistic. Second, write down the reasons why you want to change. Third, set a timescale for achieving your goals. Finally, monitor your progress by filling in a training diary. Reward your progress once you reach each mini-goal.

SUMMARY OF KEY POINTS

- The main components of a programme are the selection of exercises, ordering of exercises, number of sets and reps, rest periods, and the training intensity.
- The exercises you select for your workout depend on your specific goals and your level of experience. For strength, mass and endurance, select maximum-stimulation exercises.
- The ordering of your exercises affects the energy and effort you are able to put into the next exercise. Going from the largest to the smallest muscle groups is recommended for beginners and advanced weight trainers, while performing supersets for the same muscle group is recommended only for advanced weight trainers.
- The number of sets you perform depends on the size of the muscle group being trained, the number of muscle groups trained per session and your training experience.
- The rest period you need to leave between workouts depends on the intensity and duration of your workout, your training experience, and your diet.
- You can increase your training and intensity by increasing the amount of weight, number of sets or repetitions, number of exercises, or reducing rest intervals between sets.
- Maximum strength is developed using heavy weights and low-repetition sets, typically 2–6 sets of 6 or fewer repetitions.
- Power is developed by performing a compound exercise explosively – typically 5 sets of 1–5 repetitions using moderate weights (75–85 per cent 1RM).
- Muscle size (hypertrophy) is best developed using moderate to heavy weights (67–85 per cent 1RM) and moderate repetition sets, typically 6–12 repetitions for 3–6 sets.
- Muscular endurance is developed by using lighter weights, higher repetitions (12 or more) and minimal rest intervals (typically less than 30 seconds).
- Failure to make progress is often due to a combination of reasons centred on programme design, training technique and goal-setting.
- Slow gains may be the result of poor programme design – for example, choosing inappropriate exercises, performing too many reps or sets, or taking inadequate rest.
- A lack of programme progression leads to training plateaus as muscles require continual changes in stimulus to grow.
- Progression can be achieved by changing any one of the following variables: the number of reps and sets; the type and order of exercises; the training tempo and training split.
- Poor technique and incomplete ROM are common faults that will reduce your gains.
- Failure to set specific goals and make a plan of action sets you up for failure.

HOW TO GET STARTED

5

There are several important decisions you need to make before embarking on a weights programme, not least where you are going to train, what equipment you will use and what workout gear you will need. This chapter covers these key areas and helps you make the right decisions for you.

HOME VS GYM TRAINING

The decision whether to join a gym or train at home will depend on your fitness goals and the constraints of your lifestyle. Ask yourself the following questions:

- What are your fitness goals?
- How much time can you spend training?
- How much money do you want to spend?
- How good are you at motivating yourself?
- How sociable are you?
- How good are you at achieving your goals?
- How far are you prepared to travel to a gym?

Table 5.1 summarises the advantages and disadvantages of training at home or in a gym.

DESIGNING YOUR HOME GYM

Create a designated area in your home to train in – a basement workout room, the garage. It should be somewhere that provides a good atmosphere for training, similar to a gym.

- Buy good-quality equipment – try it out before you buy.
- Keep this space as a home gym – don't use it for storage.
- Create a gym atmosphere – play music, hang mirrors and pictures on the wall and put rubber mats on the floor to prevent damage from the weights.
- Make your home gym a 'real' gym.

CHECKLIST FOR FINDING A GOOD GYM

If, however, you decide you would like to join a gym, you will need to consider the following.

Travelling distance and time

Decide how far you are prepared to travel. If the journey takes you more than 15–20 minutes you are unlikely to visit the gym regularly once the initial novelty has worn off.

Type of equipment

Is there a good range of equipment to suit your needs? If you want to build mass, you will need plenty of free weights (see below), benches and racks. If you are more interested in general fitness and toning, you may prefer a greater range of machines and lighter free weights.

Table 5.1	The pros and cons of training at home and at the gym		
GYM		**HOME**	
Advantages	**Disadvantages**	**Advantages**	**Disadvantages**
• Greater variety of equipment, including free weights, machines and cardiovascular equipment • Instructors on hand to ensure that you are training correctly, offering advice and helping you develop your training programme • More motivating to train with other people and in a sociable club atmosphere • Spotter or training partners allow you to train harder and reduce the risk of injury or accidents • You may have access to other fitness facilities that would complement your strength training, such as a swimming pool and fitness classes	• Membership fees can be expensive, although once you've paid you may be more motivated to stick to your programme and less likely to skip workouts • Overcrowding, particularly during peak times, may be a problem • More time-consuming to travel to a gym	• You are training in the privacy of your own home • You can train when you like • You don't have to travel to the gym, so it can save time	• Initial outlay for home gym equipment can be expensive • Your budget and available space will probably limit you to the basics • Your initial enthusiasm may wear off fast and, unless you set aside specific times to work out, you can always find other things to do instead • Unless you train with a partner or personal trainer, it can be difficult to motivate yourself and push yourself hard enough to achieve significant gains • Greater risk of accident or injury unless training with a partner or personal trainer

Standard and safety of equipment

Good equipment does not need to be state-of-the-art shiny machinery. Check that the equipment is well maintained with no broken or loose attachments, and that it is cleaned and tested regularly.

Gym layout

The gym should be well ventilated and well laid out, with enough space between equipment to prevent accidents and overcrowding.

Atmosphere and motivation

The gym environment should be motivating for you as an individual. Some gyms are very busy and noisy, others are quieter; it is important to train in an atmosphere that suits your temperament. Try to get an idea of the type of members who train there – are they serious bodybuilders or general fitness trainers, sociable or quiet?

Instruction

Check that the instructors are professionally qualified. Most instructors in the UK will have a certificate (minimum NVQ Level 2) in fitness training or resistance training, or hold a degree in sports science or a related subject.

Arrange a trial workout

Most gyms will be happy to arrange a trial workout. Arrange to visit at the same time as you plan to exercise so you can see whether the gym becomes overcrowded and if you will need to queue for equipment.

Cost

Make sure you find out the true cost of joining a gym. Some require an initial non-refundable joining fee, plus an annual or monthly membership subscription. Others may allow you to pay for each workout – multiply this by the number of times you intend to train per year. Also make sure you are clear about what the membership buys you, whether you need to pay extra for other facilities, and ask about different payment methods. Find out whether any discounts are available (e.g. off-peak membership).

FREE WEIGHTS VS MACHINES

Free weights and machines offer different benefits and can both be included in a strength training programme.

THE CASE FOR FREE WEIGHTS

When you perform an exercise with free weights, you not only use the specific muscles involved in the lift (the prime movers) but the rest of the body gets involved too. You have to work to balance and control the weight using another set of muscles that acts to stabilise your body and keep the bar or dumbbells in the correct trajectory. This helps develop greater coordination skills and facilitates greater strength development.

Machines, on the other hand, keep the weight in only one trajectory so fewer muscles and motor units are recruited.

Since machines lock you into a fixed plane of movement, they reduce the contribution of the stabiliser muscles and so require less balance and skill to perform an exercise. This may be advantageous for beginners with poor motor skills, and poor muscle and postural awareness, but as muscles receive less stimulation so strength and size gains will be smaller.

Another problem with machines is that they do not accommodate the natural leverage of the body. Everyone has a unique set of levers, which will not exactly fit a machine. The resistance cams are set to match the strength curves of the 'average' person, which means that for everyone else the heaviest resistance occurs at inappropriate angles. A lower weight usually has to be selected in order to complete the movement correctly. Result: slower gains in strength and size.

Several different variations of the same exercise may be performed with free weights – e.g. bench presses with different grip widths or with the bench adjusted to different angles – thus making many different exercises possible. Machines offer fewer variations, thus potentially compromising overall development.

THE CASE FOR MACHINES

Machines and cables are good for isolating muscles and are generally safer than free weights, particularly when training without a partner or spotter: the weight stack can be returned to the starting position if you fail to complete a full repetition. Dumbbells and barbells can be dropped and plates can become unsecured.

Machines are good for beginners, for developing the basic motor skills and body awareness needed to control a movement. Once you have acquired this confidence, you can include more free-weight exercises in your routine.

WORKOUT ACCESSORIES

TRAINING GLOVES

Training gloves give your palms just enough padding to improve your grip of the bar or dumbbells, and prevent calluses and blisters from forming on your hands. They are useful for any pressing, pulling or curling movement.

Using gloves is also more hygienic than using bare hands – resistance training apparatus can be sweaty and dirty, and an ideal breeding place for germs.

TRAINING BELT

A training belt is thought to provide extra support for the lower back. However, it is only advantageous when using maximal weights, and then only for certain exercises performed vertically which place considerable stress on the vertebrae, such as heavy squats and dead lifts. It helps under these circumstances by increasing abdominal wall pressure. The tighter the belt, the greater the abdominal pressure against the spine, which thereby helps to protect the discs and other vulnerable structures. The abdominal wall should be drawn in towards the spine when lifting with a belt rather than being pushed out against it.

Do not use a belt for lighter exercises or if you have a lower-back injury or weakness. Using a belt for any other exercises in your workout can stimulate incorrect movement of the abdominal wall, leading to a weakening of the abdominal muscles.

STRAPS

Grip failure can be a limiting factor in pulling movements such as chins, seated rows and lat pull-downs. Up to a point, training without straps will help to develop the forearm muscles and strengthen your grip. However, once your grip strength starts to limit the amount of weight you can use or reduce the number of reps you can do, you should use straps. They will help you to focus on the muscle you are training and reduce the involvement of the limiting muscles. Straps are therefore advantageous for most back exercises and pulling movements performed with heavy weights.

KNEE WRAPS

Knee wraps can help support the knee joint during heavy leg exercises such as dead lifts and squats because they assist the ligaments in stabilising the joint. As with training belts, do not rely on wraps if you have a knee injury or to help you lift heavier weights than your strength allows. They are best used for maximal weights (e.g. twice your body weight) rather than as a crutch for lighter sets.

GOAL-SETTING

The key to success in any exercise programme is setting your goals and focusing your mind on reaching them. How well and how fast you achieve your goals depends on how motivated you are. But first you need to set clear goals and work out a plan to measure your success.

HOW TO SET GOALS

Goals should be **SMART**:

S = specific
M = measurable
A = agreed
R = realistic
T = time scaled

Specific

Write down exactly what you want to achieve from your training programme. Avoid vague statements such as 'tone up' or 'get stronger' as these will not focus your mind on achieving a particular result. Your goals could include details of how much lean weight you wish to gain and how much fat you wish to lose. For example, 'lose 5 kg fat and gain 3 kg muscle'. You could also write down your desired body measurements, or how much weight you wish to lift on specific exercises such as the bench press, squat and dead lift.

To help you crystallise your goals, write down the reasons why you want to improve – whether it is increased muscle size, a more symmetrical physique, better sports performance or more energy. Go beyond the superficial reasons and find the inner motivations that are driving your goals. Research shows that it is the internal motivators that really drive us to success.

Measurable

You need to be able to measure your progress. Long-term goals can be broader in scope, but short-term goals must be quite specific. Indeed, the specific goals above could be in terms of your body weight, body fat measurements, girth measurements or the amount of weight lifted, which are clearly measurable too. For example, you may wish to set a goal of 60 kg for your maximal bench press, or reduce your body fat by 5 per cent. To help monitor your progress, photocopy the training log in Figure 5.1 to record the exact weight lifted, the number of repetitions and the number of sets completed at each workout, and use them to check what you have achieved each week against your long-term goal. Keep your training records for future reference as well. In the example given in Figure 5.1 for the bench press, 40/15 would mean 15 repetitions (reps) with 40 kg.

Agreed

Ideally, discuss and agree your goals with someone – a qualified instructor, your partner, or a friend. The most important thing is committing your goals to paper; this signals a commitment to change. Write them in the form of a personal mission statement; then sign and date what you have written. Better still, ask someone else to sign the document as a witness, as you would with a contract. Then place a copy somewhere you can see it each day, such as on your desk or on a bulletin board. The goals will constantly remind you that they are waiting to be achieved. If you do not commit your goals to paper, then it is unlikely that you'll be able to commit to the work necessary to make them happen. Like a legal contract, this technique will keep your mind focused.

Exercise	Date	Date	Date	Date	Date	Date	Date
	Set (kg/reps)	Set (kg/reps)	Set (kg/reps)	Set (kg/reps)	Set (kg/reps)	Set (kg/reps)	Set (kg/reps)

*Note: only advanced weight trainers should include 5 sets of any given exercise in their programme.

Figure 5.1 Training log

Realistic

The goals should be realistic – attainable for your body size, natural shape and lifestyle. There's nothing wrong with aiming for the top but, at the same time, be realistic. If it's a gold medal you seek, study the path others have taken to achieve that goal and check it against your starting point, and how much time and energy you have to follow a similar path.

Time scaled

Set a clear time scale for reaching your goals. Decide on a deadline – this prompts action and sets your plan in motion. Without a clear deadline, it's easy to put off starting your programme and you may end up never achieving your goals.

Once you have fixed your major goals, set mini-goals, which can be reached in a relatively short period of time (such as 12 weeks), and long-term goals, which can be reached over, say, a year. You may even find it helpful to break up each 12-week goal into distinct segments and focus on the progress you make each week. For example, if your goal is to reduce your body fat percentage from 30 per cent to 20 per cent, break this down into smaller goals spread out over the course of several weeks. You could aim to achieve 24 per cent body fat within 12 weeks, but aim to reduce your body fat by 1 per cent every 2 weeks. Then aim to achieve 20 per cent within the next 12 weeks by reducing your body fat by 1 per cent every 3 weeks.

Set out a programme of activities or steps that you need to complete in order to reach each goal. These steps may include resistance training 3 times a week, eating six balanced meals a day, and doing a cardio workout 3 times a week first thing in the morning. The key is to make sure each step is specific, realistic and achievable.

MOTIVATION

VISUALISE SUCCESS

The ability to visualise success is one of the most effective tools of high-achievers. Use imagery to help you stick to your programme. Have a clear mental picture of how you will look or how you will perform at the end. Role models can help to motivate you. Pick one with a similar natural body type, shape and size as you – that way, you know you can achieve your goals and won't lose heart if you don't look similar to them, or perform like them, after a period of training. You may find it helpful to cut out pictures from a magazine and keep these with your training log.

If you are finding it difficult to motivate yourself for a workout, visualise yourself successfully completing it. Use as many senses as possible – the sight of the gym, the sounds around you. See yourself loading the weights on the bar, see yourself completing each repetition, and hear the sound of voices or music in the gym.

CREATE A MOTIVATING ENVIRONMENT

Training should give you a buzz and make you feel good about yourself. If you have to force yourself to work out when your heart is not in it, you will not train hard enough to make sufficient gains, and you are more likely to give up.

Make sure you choose the right training environment (see also p. xx) and consider enlisting the help of a training partner (see below). That way, training will become a satisfying and empowering experience that you look forward to rather than dread.

WORK OUT WITH A PARTNER

Training with someone else will increase your motivation, make training more enjoyable, allow you to train harder, decrease the chances of you skipping workouts, and help you to stick to your training programme. Choose someone with similar goals to your own but not necessarily the same ability. The important thing is that you can motivate each other.

MONITOR YOUR PROGRESS

Keep a training and nutrition diary to record your progress. Remember, achieving your goals will not happen overnight. It comes after weeks or months of committed effort. Monitor your progress on a regular basis so you can check that your actions are producing the results you want. If they are not, you need to take the necessary steps to get back on track. Training and nutrition diaries can be great motivators during workouts. Look back over your notes at the end of each week. If your performance matches your goals, reward yourself.

Use a notebook to record the following details:

- details of each exercise, sets, reps and how much weight you used (using an exercise log like that in Figure 5.1)
- how you felt before and after each workout
- what and how much you ate each day
- details of any other exercise you took
- your body measurements, including percentage body fat (see 'Measuring your body fat percentage' in the accompanying box), waist, chest, hip, leg and arm circumference measurements, or just how snugly your clothes fit (see

the 'Measurement log' in Table 5.2; you may wish to photocopy this or redraw it so that you can fill in your details).

Measuring your body fat percentage

Skinfold calipers and body fat monitors are the easiest and most accessible methods for estimating body fat.

- Skinfold calipers: calibrated calipers measure the layer of fat beneath the skin at a number of specific sites on the body, usually the biceps, triceps, below the shoulder blades and above the hip bone. The sum of the skinfolds is used in a simple equation to estimate your body fat percentage. The accuracy of this method depends almost entirely on the skill of the tester, as well as the precision of the calipers.
- Body fat monitor: this works on the principle of bioelectrical impedance. An electrode is placed on two specific points on the body – usually on one hand and the opposite foot – and an electric current is passed through them. Body fat creates an impedance, or resistance, to the current while fat-free mass permits a greater current flow. The body fat monitor measures the impedance and then uses additional information you've provided (such as your sex and height) to calculate your percentage of fat-free mass and the percentage of body fat. The accuracy depends on hydration, skin temperature, and alcohol and food consumption. It is less accurate for very lean or obese individuals.

HOW TO GET STARTED

Table 5.2	Measurement log						
	Date	Chest	Waist	Hips	Thigh	Arm	Body fat %
Start							
Week 1							
Week 2							
Week 3							
Week 4							
Week 5							
Week 6							
Week 7							
Week 8							
Week 9							
Week 10							
Week 11							
Week 12							

Photographs taken before you start your new programme and then at intervals throughout your training will help to give you feedback on your progress. This is more objective than simply looking in the mirror.

VARY YOUR WORKOUTS

Your body adapts to a certain workload and soon stops developing. Change your workout periodically to keep your body challenged and to keep boredom at bay. When you start a strength training programme, gains are rapid but then slow down or reach a plateau. Ask your gym instructor to review or devise a more intense workout when you get in a rut. Try changing the following aspects of your programme:

- the exercises for each body part
- the split of your programme
- the order of exercises
- the weights used.

Also take a complete rest from resistance training every few months and spend a week or two doing a completely different activity.

USE A PERSONAL TRAINER

If you do not have a training partner or you need extra motivation, consider using a personal trainer either on an occasional or regular basis. A personal trainer will not only design your programme but will help keep you motivated. He or she will make sure that you are on track with your goals and that you don't skip any workouts; they will give you advice on a whole range of subjects; they will help you get more out of your training; and also allow you to train at a time that is convenient for you.

To find a personal trainer, ask friends for recommendations, or check with your gym for trainers who are qualified to NVQ Level 3 and have a qualification in personal training. Also check out trainers' references and make sure that they are insured. The Exercise Register (www. exerciseregister.org) lists fully qualified and insured trainers in the UK.

REWARD YOURSELF

Give yourself rewards when you have reached a goal, no matter how small. This could be something as simple as a star for reaching your weekly target, or a new training outfit, a trip to the theatre, a meal out, new clothes or a sports massage appointment.

SUMMARY OF KEY POINTS

- The benefits of training in a commercial gym include access to a wider range of equipment, professional instruction, greater motivation and social contact.

- A home gym offers greater privacy and convenience.
- Free weights develop better balance and co-ordination than machines, accommodate the natural leverage of the body and allow a more natural plane of movement, all facilitating greater strength development.
- Machines are safer and easier for beginners.
- Training gloves are useful for all weight trainers. Training belts should only be used for vertical exercises such as the squat when using maximal weights, and knee wraps for heavy leg exercises. Straps help to reduce the involvement of limiting muscles in certain pulling and back exercises.

It is imperative to set clear short-term and long-term goals before you embark on any fitness programme. Goals should be SMART: specific, measurable, agreed, realistic and time scaled.

Motivation can be increased by visualisation techniques, training with a partner, keeping a training log and a record of your measurements, varying your routine, using a personal trainer, rewarding your progress.

// WARMING UP

It is important to warm up before beginning your workout because:

- it helps reduce the chances of injury
- it can improve your performance.

Muscles respond better to exercise if they are properly prepared for the coming workload. Warming up increases blood flow to the muscles and lubricates the joints because the fluid surrounding them becomes less viscous and the joint can move more smoothly and efficiently. At rest, muscles receive only about 15 per cent of your total blood supply, but during exercise the requirement for fuel and oxygen increases sharply and they may need up to 80 per cent of the total blood flow to meet the demand. It takes time to reroute the blood, and this cannot be achieved efficiently if you omit the warm-up and start exercising vigorously.

Warming up also improves the elasticity of the muscles, enabling them to work harder, more efficiently and for longer before they fatigue, as well as allowing nerve impulses to be transmitted faster.

Importantly, warming up also prepares you mentally for the work ahead; it increases your arousal level and motivation. Performing 1 or 2 warm-up sets with light weights acts as a mental rehearsal and means that you can perform your subsequent heavier sets more effectively.

WARM-UP TECHNIQUES

The time taken on this part of your workout depends to a large extent on the temperature of your surroundings – the cooler the environment, the longer it will take to raise your body temperature. Your warm-up should include the following three components:

1. Light cardiovascular work (5–10 minutes) to raise your body temperature and prepare your body for more strenuous exercise. This can be done on a stationary bike, treadmill, stepper, rower or elliptical trainer. Make sure you exercise continuously for at least 5 minutes at an intensity that allows you to break into a sweat.
2. Mobilisation of the major joints – this could include movements such as arm circles, knee bends and shoulder circles, which take the joints through their full ROM. These are not stretching exercises as they are continuous and do not increase the ROM.

3. Warm-up sets with light weights and high repetitions. Never embark on your working (heavy) sets straightaway because your muscles won't be properly warmed up and you will risk injury. Start with 1 or 2 sets using very light weights – around 25–50 per cent 1RM (see p. 23) – for 15–20 repetitions to warm up the target muscles, ligaments and joints, and to rehearse the action to be performed.

TO STRETCH OR NOT TO STRETCH?

Previously it was thought that stretching before strenuous activity would help prepare the muscles for exercise and reduce the risk of injury. However, more recent research suggests that stretching before you start training is unlikely to benefit your performance or reduce the risk of injury (Shrier, 1999; Shrier & Gossal, 2000; Witvrouw *et al*, 2004). A review of studies concluded that stretching in addition to aerobic warm-up does not affect the incidence of overuse injuries (McHugh & Cosgrave, 2010).

There is no evidence either that pre-exercise stretching prevents post-exercise soreness or tenderness. Most experts believe that stretching is best kept to a minimum prior to strength and power training. An active warm-up, including the three components outlined above, is more effective.

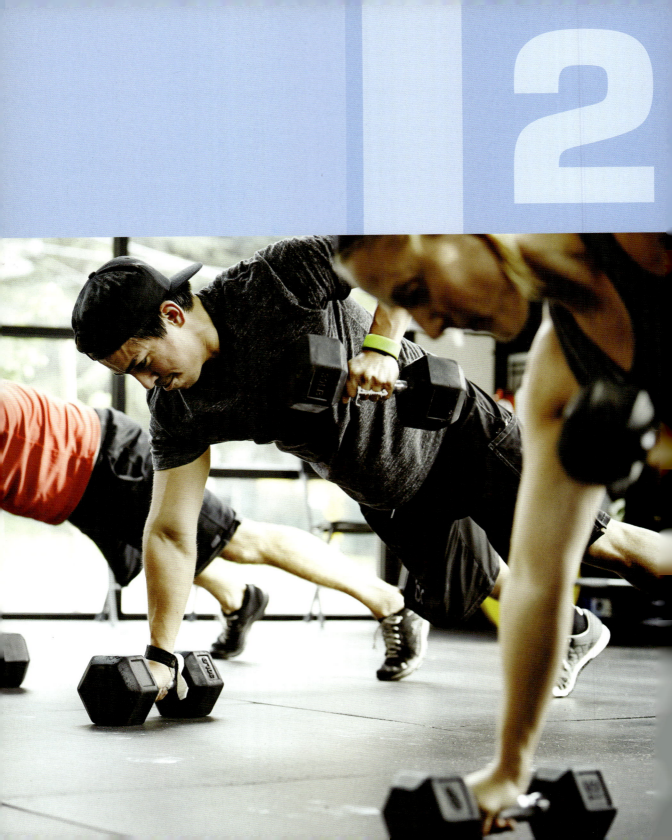

PART **TWO**

NUTRITION

Good nutrition is a crucial part of a strength training programme. Whether you want to build muscle or increase your strength, a healthy food intake will help fuel intense workouts, maximise your gains in the gym and improve your health. It will also promote recovery after training, reduce fatigue and help you achieve a healthy body composition.

Resistance exercise provides the stimulus; your diet provides the raw materials for building muscle. The idea is to stress the muscles just hard enough during your workout to break down muscle proteins and cause very small (micro) tears in the fibres. This 'damage' triggers muscle protein synthesis (MPS), or muscle growth (Rennie *et al*, 2000). When MPS exceeds muscle protein breakdown (MPB) over time, then muscle growth, or hypertrophy, occurs. After your workout, muscle proteins break down, releasing cytokines (hormone-like molecules) that signal muscle repair for up to 48 hours. These activate various pathways such as mTOR and AKT that begin the process of MPS. Short for Mammalian Target of Rapamycin, mTOR is the functioning unit that senses nutrient and oxygen levels in cells. AKT is a protein that signals cell division and growth. These pathways enable amino acids to pass from the bloodstream into the muscle cell and then get transported within the cell to where they will be assembled into new muscle proteins. Thus, these new proteins are added to the muscle fibres, making the muscle stronger and denser.

BUILD MUSCLE NOT FAT

To build muscle, you need to consume a calorie surplus. The problem is some of these excess calories will go towards the repair and growth of new muscle, and some of those calories may spill over and be stored as fat. It's possible to minimise fat gain while gaining muscle but don't expect to reduce it – you cannot build muscle and lose fat at the same time. Instead, you should prioritise your goal, i.e. build muscle or lose fat and focus on one at a time. The trick is to keep your calorie surplus high enough for muscle growth, but not so high that it results in fat storage. Follow these simple rules:

- Get your calories from real foods – it's far harder to gain fat if you focus on 'real' foods, i.e. minimally processed foods such as meat, poultry, fish, eggs, beans, lentils, nuts, seeds, fruit, vegetables, whole grains, milk, cheese, yoghurt, butter and olive oil. These foods increase satiety and reduce hunger.
- Don't go overboard with your calorie surplus – most people only need a surplus of 300–500 calories a day. Going any higher than this is likely to start a spillover and your body may store these extra calories as fat.

- Track your calories – use a calorie counter app such as myfitnesspal or a simple pad and pen to keep a daily food diary. You don't have to be very accurate, but you do need to have a good idea of your daily calorie intake.
- Train for muscle gain – an intense, effective workout routine is essential to stimulate growth and put your calorie surplus to use. If you don't follow a consistent training programme, then the extra calories you consume will turn into fat.
- Include some cardiovascular exercise – including a few short (10–20 minutes), high-intensity interval cardiovascular sessions a week is a good way to keep those unwanted fat gains under control (see page 246). This kind of exercise supports muscle growth while eliminating excess fat storage.

ESTIMATING YOUR CALORIE REQUIREMENT

The most important thing when it comes to building muscle is calories. To gain weight, you need to take in more calories than you burn. Scientists recommend increasing your usual calorie intake by 20 per cent, which works out at about 500–750 extra calories for men and 250–500 extra calories for women. These calories should come from a balanced intake of carbohydrate, protein and fat. First, you need to estimate your maintenance calories, then you need to add 20 per cent. Use one of the following methods:

1. ESTIMATION BASED ON CURRENT DIET

If your weight has been stable for several months, it can be assumed that your current daily calorie intake is roughly equivalent to your maintenance calories. To estimate your current intake, record your food and drink intake for 7 days. Be as accurate as possible, recording the exact weights of all foods and drinks consumed. Use food tables, the Internet or food labels to work out your daily calorie intake. Add up all 7 days and divide by 7 to get a daily average. To gain weight, add 20 per cent to that number (multiply by 1.2). This will be your new calorie intake to start adding muscle.

2. CALCULATION BASED ON BODY WEIGHT AND ACTIVITY

1. Estimate your resting metabolic rate (RMR) using the appropriate equation in Table 7.1.

This is the number of calories you burn at rest over 24 hours, maintaining essential functions such as respiration, digestion and brain function.

Example

For a 28-year-old 70 kg male:
RMR = (70 x 15.3) + 679 = 1750 kcal

2. Calculate the daily energy needs of your lifestyle based on your physical activity level (PAL), using the information below.

Physical activity level	Lifestyle daily energy needs
Mostly inactive or sedentary (mainly sitting)	RMR x 1.2
Moderately active (exercise 2–3 x weekly)	RMR x 1.4
Active (exercise hard, more than 3 x weekly)	RMR x 1.5
Very active (exercise hard daily)	RMR x 1.7

Multiply your RMR by your PAL to estimate your maintenance daily calorie needs:
RMR x PAL

Table 7.1	Resting metabolic rate in athletes	
Age (years)	**Men**	**Women**
10–18	(body weight in kg x 17.5) + 651	(body weight in kg x 12.2) + 746
19–30	(body weight in kg x 15.3) + 679	(body weight in kg x 14.7) + 496
31–60	(body weight in kg x 11.6) + 879	(body weight in kg x 8.7) + 829
60 + years	(body weight in kg x 13.5) + 487	(body weight in kg x 10.5) + 596

Example

For a 28-year-old 70 kg male who is moderately active (exercises 2–3 times a week):
Daily energy needs (without exercise)

    = 1750 x 1.4
    = 2450 kcal

This is roughly how many calories you burn a day to maintain your weight, assuming you have an 'average' body composition. If you have higher than average muscle mass, add 150 calories.

3. To gain weight, increase your calorie intake by 20 per cent. Multiply your maintenance calories by 1.2.

Example

For a 28-year-old 70 kg male who is moderately active (exercises 2–3 times a week):
Daily energy needs to gain weight

    = 2450 x 1.2
    = 2940 kcal

4. To lose weight, reduce your calorie intake by 15 per cent. Multiply your maintenance calories by 0.85.

Example

For a 28-year-old 70 kg male who is moderately active (exercises 2–3 times a week):
Daily energy needs to lose weight

    = 2450 x 0.85
    = 2083 kcal

Table 7.2	Calories expended during exercise	
		Kcal per hour
Sport	**Men**	**Women**
Cycling (11.2 kph)	300	234
Cycling (16 kph)	450	354
Rowing machine	480	377
Running (12 kph)	840	660
Running (16 kph)	1092	858
Swimming (crawl, 4.8 kph)	1200	942
Tennis (singles)	426	330
Resistance training	492	384

Cutting your calorie intake

To reduce your body fat, cut your calories by 15 per cent. This relatively modest decrease minimises any drop in your metabolic rate and allows you to retain your hard-earned muscle.

The problem with drastically restricting your calorie intake is that you cause your metabolic rate to slow down. This is called the 'starvation adaptation response' and means that your body stockpiles fat and calories rather than burning them for energy so that it becomes harder and harder for your body to burn fat. Your glycogen stores also quickly deplete, causing fatigue, a drop in performance, low energy levels and mounting hunger. Worse still, you end up breaking down muscle tissue as well as fat to provide fuel. On the other hand, cutting your calories by a modest 15 per cent will produce steady fat loss without sacrificing significant muscle. You can expect to lose roughly 0.5 kg fat/week, slightly more when combined with the cardiovascular training programme described in Chapter 25.

CARBOHYDRATE

Carbohydrate, in the form of muscle glycogen and blood glucose, is the major source of fuel for high-intensity strength training. If you don't eat enough carbohydrate you'll fatigue sooner (due to low muscle glycogen levels) and your muscle and strength gains will be reduced. Fat cannot fuel high-intensity all-out exercise – only carbohydrate can produce energy fast enough.

Carbohydrate is also important for muscle building because it stimulates the release of insulin – an anabolic hormone that drives protein and carbohydrates into the muscle cells, encouraging muscle building. Studies have also shown that low-carb diets tend to increase cortisol levels, and decrease testosterone and thyroid levels (Lane *et al*, 2010). In other words, a low-carbohydrate intake combined with intense training can result in protein breakdown and loss of muscle mass.

On the other hand, eating too much carbohydrate in one meal or over the course of a day may result in unwanted body fat once the body's glycogen storage capacity is exceeded. Try to listen to your body and you'll soon find the balance between too little and too much carbohydrate.

CARBOHYDRATE REQUIREMENT

Previously, sports scientists recommended that all athletes should get around 60 per cent of their calories from carbohydrate. But this doesn't take account of different exercise modes (e.g. endurance or resistance), body weights or training volumes. For strength athletes, it is more accurate to calculate carbohydrate requirement according to the muscles' needs rather than total calorie intake. Muscle glycogen is not depleted to the same extent as that of endurance athletes and there is longer recovery time between working the same muscle group. Carbohydrate needs are more accurately expressed as grams per kg of body weight and hours of training.

For most people, the amount of activity you do varies from day to day, so you will need to vary your carbohydrate intake accordingly. So, on days when you are more active, you should eat more carbohydrate; conversely, on rest days or when you do a lighter workout, you should eat correspondingly less carbohydrate.

As a rule of thumb, the longer and harder you train, the more carbohydrate you need to fuel your muscles (Rodriguez *et al*, 2009; IOC, 2011). The consensus is 3–5 g/kg body weight/day for relatively low-intensity exercise, such as brisk walking or skill-based workouts (Burke, L., 2007; Burke L. *et al*, 2011). For moderate-intensity training equating to about 1 hour per day, an intake between 5 and 7 g/kg body weight daily is recommended. Moderate- to high-intensity training up to 3 hours a day increases your requirement to 7–10 g/kg body weight. In practice, around 5–7 g/kg should be more than adequate for most people training 1–2 hours a day. Even if you're lifting heavy weights, this level will be more than enough to fuel a typical workout. Only elite endurance athletes who are in very heavy training need more than 7 g/kg on a daily basis. Table 7.3 gives guidelines for daily carbohydrate intake for different types and duration of training programmes.

Example

For a 70 kg male training at a moderate intensity for 1 hour a day:

Carbohydrate needs = (70 x 5)–(70 x 7)
= 350–490 g/day

Table 7.3	How much carbohydrate?			
Activity level	Recommended carbohydrate intake g/kg body weight/day	carbohydrate/day for a 50 kg person	carbohydrate/day for a 60 kg person	carbohydrate/day for a 70 kg person
Very light training (low-intensity or skill-based exercise)	3–5 g	150–250 g	180–300 g	210–350 g
Moderate-intensity training (approx 1 h/day)	5–7 g	250–350 g	300–420 g	350–490 g
Moderate- to high-intensity training (1–3 h/day)	7–10 g	350–500 g	420–600 g	490–700 g
Very high-intensity training (> 4 h/day)	10–12 g	500–600 g	600–720 g	700–840 g

(Source: Burke, L., 2007; Burke L. *et al*, 2011.)

However, this is only a guideline and you should adjust this according to your specific training goals, how active you are during the rest of the day, and how you feel during and after training. For example, if you want to lose weight, you should eat less than this amount.

Table 7.4 gives the carbohydrate content of various foods but you can also get an idea of your carbohydrate intake by checking the labels of foods or using the free online database http://www.food-database.co.uk/ for the amounts of carbs in various foods.

WHICH CARBOHYDRATES?

Choose mostly fibre-rich carbohydrates like potatoes, bread, porridge, rice, pasta, fruit, beans and lentils. Honey, dried fruit and fruit juice are denser sources of carbohydrates and make it easier to reach your daily carbohydrate needs if you want to gain weight or have a fast metabolism. If you want to prevent weight gain or lose weight, focus mainly on unprocessed fibre-rich carbohydrate foods, which are more filling.

Low-GI diets are beneficial for strength trainers as well as the general population. They can help control blood sugar levels, appetite and body weight, lower blood fats, reduce the risk of diabetes and heart disease, and control body weight. For strength trainers a low-GI daily diet is particularly important for encouraging glycogen recovery between workouts. It produces steadier blood glucose and insulin levels, which facilitates a steady uptake of glucose by the muscle cells for glycogen storage, and minimises the conversion of blood glucose into body fat.

The best way to plan a low-GI diet is to balance each meal by including:

- a source of protein (e.g. meat, poultry, fish, beans, lentils, eggs, cheese or milk)
- a fibre-rich carbohydrate (e.g. potatoes, wholegrain rice, bread or pasta)

Table 7.4	The carbohydrate content of different foods	
Food	**Energy (kcal)**	**Carbohydrate (g)**
Apples (one, 100 g)	47	12
Baked beans (200 g)	162	30
Bananas (one, 100 g)	95	23
Biscuits (one, 15 g)	70	10
Bran flakes (40 g)	132	29
Bread (1 slice, 35 g)	80	15
Cereal bar (one, 30 g)	140	18
Flapjacks (one, 70 g)	345	44
Jam or honey (15 g)	40	10
Milk, semi-skimmed (300 ml)	138	14
Oatcakes (one, 13 g)	54	8
Orange juice (200 ml)	72	18
Pasta (85 g raw weight)	196	64
Pitta bread (one, 60 g)	160	34
Porridge (200 g)	166	23
Potatoes (200 g)	150	34
Rice (85 g raw weight)	303	69
Roll (one, 50 g)	120	22
Shreddies (40 g)	138	31
Sweetcorn (80 g)	89	16
Weetabix (two, 40 g)	141	30
Yoghurt (1 pot, 150 g)	117	21

The glycaemic index

The glycaemic index (GI) is a measure of how quickly your blood glucose will rise after eating a portion of food containing 50 g of carbohydrate. All foods containing carbohydrate are ranked on an index from 0 to 100 relative to pure glucose, which has the highest GI value of 100. Thus, high-GI foods produce a relatively rapid rise in blood glucose and low-GI foods produce a slower, more sustained rise in blood glucose. The Table on pp. 66–7 shows the GIs of various foods, divided into high-, medium- and low-GI foods.

According to this index, many complex carbohydrates – such as potatoes, bread and rice – give a quick rise in blood glucose, while many simple carbohydrates – such as fruit – give a slower rise. It is important to realise, however, that the GI values relate to single foods being consumed. When two or more foods are eaten together, the GI changes. High-GI foods eaten with protein or fat moderate the glucose response, so the GI values only count for single foods. For example, potatoes cause a relatively rapid blood glucose rise. But if you eat potatoes with a high-protein food (e.g. tuna) or a high-fat food (e.g. butter), the GI will be lower and so your blood glucose will rise more slowly.

BUILD MUSCLE NOT FAT

- vegetables or salad
- a little fat (e.g. olive oil, nuts, butter).

If you want to eat high-GI foods, eat them with fats and protein to lower the GI of the meal.

Eat high-GI foods or drinks immediately before, during (if exercising for more than an hour) and immediately after training. These help raise blood glucose quickly so can help increase endurance and speed recovery.

The Glycaemic Index (GI) of foods

Low GI foods
Low GI (< 55)

Food	GI	Food	GI
Peanuts	14	All-Bran	42
Fructose	19	Orange	42
Cherries	22	Peach	42
Grapefruit	25	Milk chocolate	43
Lentils (red)	26	Muffin, apple	44
Whole milk	27	Sponge cake	46
Chickpeas	28	Grapes	46
Red kidney beans	28	Pineapple juice	46
Lentils (green/brown)	30	Macaroni	47
Butter beans	31	Carrots	47
Apricots (dried)	31	Bulgur wheat	48
Meal replacement bar	31	Peas	48
Skimmed milk	32	Baked beans	48
Protein shake	32	Muesli	49
Fruit yoghurt (low fat)	33	Rye bread	50
Chocolate milk	34	Mango	51
Custard	35	Strawberry jam	51
Plain yoghurt (low fat)	36	Banana	52
Spaghetti	38	Orange juice	52
Apples	38	Kiwi fruit	53
Tinned peaches – tinned in fruit juice	38	Buckwheat	54
Pear	38	Sweetcorn	54
Yoghurt drink	38	Crisps	54
Protein bar	38	Muesli (Alpen)	55
Plum	39	Honey	55
Apple juice	40	Brown rice	55
Strawberries	40		

Moderate GI foods
Moderate GI (56–69)

Food	GI	Food	GI
Boiled potato (old)	56	Energy bar	56
Sultanas	56	Pitta bread	57

Apricots	57	White rice	64
Porridge	58	Shortbread	64
Basmati rice	58	Raisins	64
Squash (diluted)	58	Couscous	65
Digestive biscuits	59	Cantaloupe melon	65
Pineapple	59	Mars bar	65
Pizza	60	Instant porridge	66
Ice cream	61	Croissant	67
Sweet potato	61	Sucrose	68
Muesli bar	61	Weetabix	74
Tortillas/corn chips	63	Shredded Wheat	75
High GI foods			
High GI (> 70)			
White bread	70	Mashed potato	74
Millet	71	Chips	75
Wholemeal bread	71	Rice cakes	78
Bagel	72	Gatorade	78
Breakfast cereal bar (crunchy nut cornflakes)	72	Cornflakes	81
		Rice Krispies	82
Watermelon	72	Baked potato	85
Cheerios	74	French baguette	95
Bran flakes	74	Lucozade ™	95

Adapted with permission from *The American Journal of Clinical Nutrition* © *Am. J. Clin. Nutr.* American Society for Nutrition (Foster-Powell *et al*, 2002)

PROTEIN

Protein is important for muscle growth. The building blocks of protein, amino acids, are used for repairing and rebuilding the muscle fibres that you have damaged during your workout.

Heavy strength training stimulates an increased uptake of amino acids from the bloodstream. These amino acids are then built up into new contractile muscle proteins, actin and myosin (see p. 15). To build muscle, you must take in more protein than you excrete – i.e. be in a positive nitrogen balance. A deficient intake will result in slower gains in strength, size and mass, or even muscle loss – despite hard training. However, there is not a linear relationship between protein intake and muscle growth. Muscle growth depends not only on your protein intake but also on the intensity of your training (i.e. the training stimulus) and your genetic potential for muscle growth.

Is carbohydrate loading beneficial for bodybuilders?

Competitive bodybuilders sometimes use carbohydrate loading to increase muscle size before a competition. Whether this really is beneficial is debatable. In one study, researchers measured the muscle girth of nine male bodybuilders before and after a control and a high-carbohydrate diet (Balon et al, 1992). This carbohydrate-loading diet involved 3 days of heavy resistance training on a low-carbohydrate diet (10 per cent calories from carbohydrate), followed by 3 days of light resistance training on a high-carbohydrate diet (80 per cent calories from carbohydrate). The control diet involved the same resistance training programme but the men ate a standard diet providing the same number of calories. So what happened? Carbohydrate loading did not increase the muscle circumference in any of the bodybuilders, which suggests that it probably has no benefit after all.

Obviously, this is just a single study so its findings are not conclusive. There is plenty of anecdotal evidence from bodybuilders that carbohydrate loading before a competition improves muscle appearance. If you decide to try this regime, however, you may achieve equally good results by omitting the 3-day depletion phase and simply eating a high-carbohydrate diet for the 3 days prior to competition.

In practice, the body can adapt to variations in protein intake. Over time the body becomes more efficient in conserving it so you break down fewer muscle proteins during intense training. This is often sufficient to maintain an anabolic environment and induce muscle growth[5]. One study found that the protein requirement/kg body weight of advanced strength trainers was 40 per cent less than that of novice strength trainers.

PROTEIN REQUIREMENT

It is widely accepted that athletes have higher protein requirements than the general population (Rodriguez et al, 2009; Phillips et al, 2007; Phillips & Van Loon, 2011). The scientific consensus from the International Olympic Committee Conference on Nutrition for Sport, 2010 is an intake between 1.6 g and 1.8 g for strength and power athletes (Phillips & Van Loon, 2011). This translates to 112–126 g daily for a 70 kg person, considerably more than Guideline Daily Amount (GDA) for the general population (45 g for women and 55 g for men). This extra protein is needed to compensate for the increased breakdown of protein during exercise and to facilitate muscle repair and recovery after intense training. The majority of research shows that you don't generally need more than about 1.8 grams of protein per kilogram.

TIMING OF PROTEIN INTAKE

The timing of your protein intake around exercise is important. Studies have shown that consuming protein in the immediate post-exercise period (within 1–2 hours of training) stimulates rapid MPS and muscle hypertrophy (Hartman et al, 2007; Holm et al, 2006). However, the window for protein consumption is longer than once thought. It is now known that the anabolic effect of exercise lasts up to 24 hours so the benefits of consuming protein may extend for several hours. In other words, consuming protein immediately after training will increase MPS, but so will protein consumption at any time over the subsequent 24 hours.

It's also been shown that consuming protein before as well as after training may be beneficial (Willoughby *et al*, 2007; Tipton *et al*, 2003).

OPTIMAL POST-EXERCISE PROTEIN INTAKE

Studies suggest that 20–25 g is the optimal level for muscle growth immediately after a weights workout (Moore *et al*, 2009). When athletes consumed less than 20 g they gained less muscle; when they consumed more than this amount they experienced no further muscle gains. However, it's best to think of 20–25 g as a ballpark figure. If you weigh more than 85 kg (the weight of the athletes in the study) then you will need more; if you weigh less than 85 kg, you may need less.

For optimal protein synthesis, you should consume 0.25–0.3 g protein/kg body mass at each meal. For a 70 kg athlete, this equates to 18–21 g. Consuming less than this amount may result in a sub-optimal rate of MPS; consuming more will not produce greater strength or mass gain. Excess protein will either be used for other functions in the body or as a fuel source.

A review of studies on protein needs by researchers at McMaster University, Canada, concluded that protein should be consumed with carbohydrate in a 3 to 1 ratio after exercise (Tipton *et al*, 1999). They found that this particular protein and carbohydrate combination was more effective in promoting muscle repair and glycogen storage than protein or carbohydrate alone.

Consuming protein with carbohydrate promotes a greater release of insulin, which stimulates the transport of glucose and amino acids into muscle cells. The more insulin is present in the bloodstream, the more glucose and amino acids can be carried into the muscles

Is too much protein harmful?

Consuming more than 1.8 g protein/kg body weight/day will not make you stronger or more muscular (Lemon, 1998). In a study of strength athletes carried out at McMaster University, Canada, athletes consuming either 1.4 g/kg body weight/day or 2.3 g/kg body weight/day experienced similar increases in muscle mass (Tarnopolsky et al, 1992). Those with the higher protein intake gained no further benefits. Once your optimal intake has been reached, additional protein is not converted into muscle.

On the other hand, excess protein is unlikely to be harmful to health. Any protein that isn't needed for tissue repair and growth is partly excreted (in the form of urea) and partly used as a fuel source. Contrary to popular belief, excess protein does not harm the kidneys or cause dehydration in healthy people (Tipton & Wolfe, 2007). It does not make you fat either – eating excess calories will. Protein induces greater satiety than carbohydrate or fat, as it raises levels of satiety hormones such as glucagon, so it's actually quite difficult to eat too many calories on a high protein diet (Halton & Hu 2004).

for glycogen and protein manufacture. When protein is consumed with carbohydrate, the insulin response can nearly double that invoked by carbs alone. Insulin also blunts the rise in cortisol that would otherwise follow exercise. Cortisol suppresses protein synthesis and stimulates protein breakdown.

PROTEIN QUALITY

Milk, whey, casein, egg, meat, poultry and fish provide all the essential amino acids at levels that closely match the body's needs. Studies have shown that these types of protein stimulate muscle growth more than other types of protein.

These foods are also rich in the amino acid leucine, which has been shown to be a critical element in regulating protein manufacture in the body as well as playing a key role in muscle recovery after exercise. In combination with the other EAAs, it triggers protein manufacture, which in turn leads to increased muscle strength.

However, non-animal protein sources, such as beans, lentils, nuts, soya and (to a smaller degree) grains, also contribute amino acids to your diet and will count towards your total daily protein intake (see Table 7.5: The protein content of various foods).

Liquid forms of protein (such as milk and whey protein drinks) are particularly beneficial for MPS as they are digested and absorbed more rapidly than solid foods. Milk consumed immediately after resistance exercise has been shown to increase muscle growth and repair, reduces post-exercise muscle soreness, improves body composition and rehydrates the body better than commercial sports drinks (Elliot, 2006; Hartman *et al*, 2007; Wilkinson, 2007; Karp *et al*, 2006).

Table 7.5	The protein content of various foods
Food	**Protein (g)**
Beef sirloin steak (85 g)	21
Chicken or turkey breast (125 g)	36
Fish, e.g. salmon or haddock fillet (150 g)	30
Tuna, canned in brine (100 g)	24
Cheddar cheese, 1 slice (40 g)	10
Milk (600 ml)	21
Low fat plain yoghurt (150 g)	7
Greek plain yoghurt (150 g)	10
3 eggs (size 3)	21
Peanuts (50 g)	12
Cashews (50 g)	9
Almonds (50 g)	11
Peanut butter (20 g)	5
Pumpkin seeds (25 g)	6
Baked beans (200 g)	10
Lentils (150 g cooked)	13
Red kidney beans (150 g cooked)	10
Chickpeas (150 g cooked)	11
Soy milk alternative (600 ml)	20
Tofu burger (60 g)	5
Quorn burger (50 g)	6
Wholemeal bread (2 slices, 80 g)	7
Wholegrain rice (180 g cooked)	5
Wholegrain spaghetti (180 g cooked)	9
Quinoa (180 g uncooked)	8
Whey protein powder (25 g)	20*
Meal replacement powder (25 g)	13*
1 nutrition (sports) bar (60 g)	21*

* Values may vary depending on brand

Protein and amino acids

Proteins are made up of 20 amino acids, which are the building blocks of proteins. Nine of these are 'essential amino acids' (EAAs) – they must be supplied in the diet as the body cannot make them itself. These are histidine, isoleucine, leucine, lysine, methionine, phenylalanine, threonine, tryptophan, and valine. The remaining 11 can be made from other amino acids and are termed 'non-essential amino acids'.

Three EAAs – valine, leucine and isoleucine – are termed 'branched chain amino acids' (BCAAs), due to their branched structure. These are used as fuel for energy by muscles during intense exercise when glycogen stores are low.

Food proteins with a high EAA content in proportions closely matched to the body's requirements are said to have a high biological value (BV). This is a measure of the usefulness of a protein – that is, the proportion of the protein that can be absorbed and used for growth and repair. Eggs have the highest BV (100) of all foods.

To maximise the benefits of protein in your diet, eat a mixture of protein foods so that the shortfall of amino acids in one is complemented by higher amounts in the other. For example, combining beans and rice means that the shortfall of lysine in rice is complemented by higher amounts in the beans. Other combinations suitable for vegetarians include pasta with beans or chickpeas, toast with peanut butter, and tofu with noodles.

Milk and whey protein are particularly rich sources of leucine so both represent ideal post-workout foods for promoting muscle growth.

The optimal amount of protein needed to maximise muscle protein synthesis after exercise is 20 g, which is supplied by approximately 500–600 ml of milk. This volume of milk also provides 30 g of carbohydrate, which will help replenish muscle glycogen stores and build muscle. The type of milk (skimmed or whole milk) is unimportant as far as MPS is concerned. Milkshake, hot chocolate, latte and other coffee drinks made with milk are also suitable recovery options.

FAT

Fat is important fuel for the body as well as being crucial for health. It is made up of fatty acids, which contribute to the structure and proper functioning of body cells. It also helps absorb and transport the fat-soluble vitamins A, D, E and K, is a source of the essential omega-3 and omega-6 polyunsaturated fatty acids, and plays a vital role in the manufacture of the muscle-building hormone testosterone. High testosterone levels stimulate muscle growth and increase strength. Studies have shown that higher fat diets (40 per cent calories from fat) can boost testosterone levels (Dorgan *et al*, 1996). On the other hand, low-fat diets (less than 20 per cent calories from fat) reduce the body's production of testosterone (Hamalainen *et al*, 1983). Fat may also help to increase levels of insulin-like growth factor (IGF-1), a key hormone that stimulates muscle growth and increases strength. Low-fat diets have been shown to lower IGF-1 levels by 20 per cent (Ngo *et al*, 2002).

Although fat provides more calories per gram compared with carbohydrate or protein, it is not necessarily fattening nor should be eliminated if you're trying to lose weight. Fat is more satiating than carbohydrate, which means it gives the body the feeling of being full and therefore helps satisfy your appetite. Including moderate amounts of natural fats in the diet can help control your appetite.

FAT REQUIREMENT

The IOC makes no specific recommendation for fat (IOC, 2011), although the ACSM suggests an intake between 20 and 35 per cent of total calories (Rodriguez *et al*, 2009). Eating too little fat puts you at risk of a deficient intake of fat-soluble vitamins A, D and E and essential fatty acids.

Given the important role of fat in testosterone and IGF-1 production, it would be reasonable to aim for an intake at the top end of this range if you want to build muscle at the optimal rate.

The best way to check that your fat intake lies within this range is to calculate your calorie, carbohydrate and protein requirement (using the methods already described in this chapter). Your fat intake is the balance left once you have subtracted the carbohydrate and protein calories from your total daily calorie intake. Use the following calculation:

Carbohydrate calories = g carbohydrate x 4
Protein calories = g protein x 4
Fat calories = total daily calories – carbohydrate
    calories – protein calories
g fat = fat calories ÷ 9

So, for example, a 70 kg athlete who consumes 2450 kcal, 350 g carbohydrate (5 g/kg body weight) and 112 g protein (1.6 g/kg body weight):

Carbohydrate calories = 350 x 4 = 1400
Protein calories = 112 x 4 = 448
Fat calories = 2450 – 1400 – 448 = 602
g fat = 602 ÷ 9 = 67 g

THE DIFFERENT TYPES OF FATS

Fats (or triglycerides) found in food are made up of a glycerol 'backbone' with three fatty acids attached. Each fatty acid is a chain of carbon and hydrogen atoms and these can be classified as either saturated, monounsaturated or poly-unsaturated according to the number of double bonds it contains:

- Saturated fats contain no double bonds.
- Monounsaturated fats contain one double bond.
- Polyunsaturated fats contain two or more double bonds.

Saturated fats

Saturated fats are found in all fats but higher amounts are present in animal fats and products made with them. Main sources include meat, milk, cheese and yoghurt, butter, lard, coconut oil, palm oil and palm kernel oil (often listed as 'vegetable fat' on food labels), and eggs (yolk).

The evidence linking diets high in saturated fats with heart disease is less convincing than once thought. A scientific review of 72 studies (part funded by the British Heart Foundation) involving more than 600,000 people found no significant link between saturated fat and heart disease. It appears that the saturated fats in dairy products raise only one subtype (benign) of LDL cholesterol. However, this doesn't give you the green light to go ahead and eat as much meat and butter as you want – these foods in excess can still be harmful to health, increasing total and LDL cholesterol.

Monounsaturated fats

Monounsaturated fats are also found in all fats. Main sources include olive oil, rapeseed oil, avocados, nuts, nut butters and seeds.

Eating a diet that is moderate in total fat but rich in monounsaturated fats (such as the traditional Mediterranean diet) is thought to be healthier than low-fat diets, reducing the risk of heart disease and stroke.

Polyunsaturated fats

Main sources of polyunsaturated fats include vegetable and seed oils, such as sunflower, corn and safflower oil, as well as margarines, spreads and products made with them.

Two types of polyunsaturated fats – the omega-3 and omega-6 fatty acids – are called essential fatty acids, meaning that you need them in your diet because the body cannot produce them. Both are extremely important for maintaining the correct structure of cell membranes in the body.

ESSENTIAL FATS

The two essential fatty acids – linoleic acid and alpha-linolenic acid – are vital to your health and cannot be made in the body. When you eat linoleic acid, your body converts it into a number of other fatty acids, including gamma-linolenic acid (GLA) and docosapentaenoic acid (DPA).

Linoleic acid and its derivative fatty acids are called omega-6 fatty acids (there is a rigid link, or 'double bond', on the sixth carbon atom in the fatty acid chain). When you eat alpha-linolenic acid, your body converts it into eicosapentaenoic acid (EPA) and docosahexaenoic acid (DHA), and these are called omega-3 fatty acids (the rigid link occurs on the third carbon atom).

Omega-3 fatty acids

These fats are necessary for proper functioning of the brain, regulating hormones, for the immune system and blood flow. Omega-3 fatty acids protect against heart disease and stroke and, according to recent research, may also help improve brain function, prevent Alzheimer's disease, treat depression, and help improve the behaviour of children with dyslexia, dyspraxia and ADHD. For regular exercisers, omega-3s increase the delivery of oxygen to muscles, and improve aerobic capacity and endurance. They also help to speed up recovery and reduce inflammation and joint stiffness. Main sources include: oily fish, such as sardines, mackerel, salmon, fresh tuna, trout, herring, walnuts and walnut oil, pumpkin seeds and pumpkinseed oil, flaxseeds and flaxseed oil, dark green leafy vegetables, rapeseed oil and omega-3 enriched eggs.

Omega-6 fatty acids

Omega-6s are more widely found in foods than omega-3s. For this reason, most people currently eat too much omega-6 in relation to omega-3, which results in an imbalance of prostaglandins (hormone-like chemicals responsible for controlling blood clotting, inflammation and the immune system). It is thought that the average diet used to contain a ratio of 1:1 but over the last 100 years or so this has increased to 10:1 or even 20:1 due to an increased intake of processed foods.

Excessive levels of omega-6 (or a deficiency of omega-3) can lead to a pro-inflammatory state, which has been linked to a number of conditions including cardiovascular disease, arthritis, stroke and cancer.

HOW MUCH?

The UK government recommends 450–900 mg of the long-chain EPA and DHA per day, which can be met with one portion (140 g) of oily fish per week or one tablespoon of an omega-3-rich oil daily, which will provide around 2–3 g EPA and DHA. The omega-3 content of various foods is shown in Table 7.6.

NUTRIENT TIMING

Eating a low-GI meal 2–4 hours before training will produce a more gradual release of energy, help maintain blood sugar levels during your workout, and spare muscle glycogen. Porridge, cereal with milk, a chicken or cheese sandwich, a jacket potato with beans, or pasta with tuna are suitable pre-workout meals. Combining carbohydrate with protein and/or fat gives a slower burn than carbohydrate alone. If your last meal was more than 4 hours before your workout, have a small carbohydrate-rich snack – a banana, a handful of dried fruit, a fruit smoothie or a granola or oat-based bar – about an hour before your workout to boost blood sugar levels.

Table 7.6	Sources of omega-3 fatty acids		
Food	**Omega-3 fatty acids: g/100 g**	**Portion size**	**Omega-3 fatty acids: g/portion**
Salmon	2.5 g	100 g	2.5 g
Mackerel	2.8 g	160 g	4.5 g
Sardines, tinned	2.0 g	100 g	2.0 g
Trout	1.3 g	230 g	2.9 g
Tuna, canned in oil, drained	1.1 g	100 g	1.1 g
Cod liver oil	24 g	1 tsp (5 ml)	1.2 g
Flaxseed oil	57 g	1 tbsp (15ml)	8.0 g
Flaxseeds, ground	16 g	1 tbsp (24 g)	3.8 g
Rapeseed oil	9.6 g	1 tbsp (15ml)	1.3 g
Walnuts	7.5 g	1 tbsp (28 g)	2.6 g
Walnut oil	11.5 g	1 tbsp (15ml)	1.6 g
Peanuts	0.4 g	50 g	0.2 g
Broccoli	1.3 g	3 tbsp (125 g)	1.3 g
Pumpkin seeds	8.5 g	2 tbsp (25 g)	2.1 g
Omega-3 eggs		1 egg	0.7 g
Typical omega-3 supplement		8 capsules	0.5 g

Do workouts on an empty stomach burn more fat?

If fat loss is your main goal, exercising on an empty stomach when blood sugar and insulin levels are low may encourage your body to burn slightly more fat for fuel. However, it does not necessarily mean that you burn more calories or lose more body fat. If you exercise with low muscle glycogen levels, you may fatigue sooner and/or reduce your exercise intensity, doing fewer reps or sets or using lighter weights. In other words, you could end up burning fewer calories and less body fat! Worse, you could end up losing hard-earned muscle as you start burning protein, as well as fat, for fuel!

Although most of the research on pre-exercise meals has been carried out with endurance athletes, it seems that consuming approximately 1 g carbohydrate/kg body weight about an hour before exercise helps you keep going significantly longer than consuming nothing.

For most workouts lasting less than 1 hour, there is little benefit to be gained from consumed additional carbohydrate, whether in liquid or solid form. However, for workouts lasting longer than 1 hour, evidence from studies with endurance athletes suggests that consuming carbohydrate maintains blood sugar levels, delays fatigue, and improves endurance and performance (Burke *et al*, 2011). A few studies also suggest that consuming a carbohydrate/protein drink during and immediately after a strenuous weights workout lasting 45–60 minutes may encourage faster muscle growth, delay fatigue and give you more

energy to perform those last few sets (Fahey *et al*, 1993; Conley & Stone, 1996). It may also reduce the risk of excessive protein (muscle) breakdown during the latter stages of your workout.

However, if you wish to lose body fat or prevent fat gain, be aware that many commercial energy drinks are high in calories. If you drink too much, you could end up taking in more calories than you burn off!

Studies have shown that consuming carbohydrate within 2 hours of exercise speeds glycogen recovery and improves performance the next day (Ivy *et al*, 1988; Baker *et al*, 1994).

Combining carbohydrate with protein seems to be a more effective strategy for replenishing glycogen than consuming carbohydrate alone (Zawadski *et al*, 1992; Tarnopolsky *et al*, 1997). Protein combined with carbohydrate stimulates a greater release of insulin, which promotes faster uptake of glucose by the muscle cells and faster glycogen storage.

EATING FOR WEIGHT GAIN

Lean weight gain can be achieved by combining a consistent resistance training programme with a balanced diet. Resistance training provides the stimulus for muscle growth while your diet should provide sufficient energy (calories) and nutrients to enable your muscles to grow at the optimal rate. One without the other will result in minimal lean weight gain.

To gain lean weight at the optimal rate you need to consume approximately 20 per cent more calories than you need for maintenance. This cannot be stressed too much. These additional calories should come from a balanced ratio of carbohydrate, protein and fat. For example,

Post-workout snacks

The following options provide around 20 g of high-quality protein:

- 600 ml milk. Any type of milk will provide the protein needed to maximise muscle adaptation after strength and power training. It also contains the optimal amount of the branched chain amino acid leucine to promote muscle building after exercise.
- 500 ml yoghurt and fruit milkshake. Use 500 ml of milk plus yoghurt and fresh fruit (in general, bananas, strawberries, pears, mango and pineapple give the best results) for an excellent mixture of protein, carbohydrate and those all-important antioxidants.
- 450 ml yoghurt. Choose plain yoghurt after a strength workout, or fruit yoghurt after an endurance session lasting an hour or more. Both contain high-quality proteins that will accelerate muscle repair; fruit yoghurt has added sugar so it has the ideal 3 to 1 carbohydrate to protein ratio for speedy glycogen refuelling.
- 330–500 ml whey protein shake. Shakes made up with milk or water are an easy and convenient mini-meal in a glass. Opt for one containing 20 g protein. Powders and ready-to-drink versions generally contain a balanced mixture of carbohydrate (usually as maltodextrin and sugar), protein (usually whey), vitamins and minerals.
- 50 g of almonds or cashews plus 250 ml yoghurt – nuts provide not only 10 g of protein but also B vitamins, vitamin E, iron, zinc, phytonutrients and fibre. Yoghurt supplies another 10 g of protein. The fat in the nuts may reduce insulin a little, but will not affect muscle building.
- 250 ml strained Greek yoghurt. This is also perfect after a strength workout, because strained Greek yoghurt is more concentrated, containing about twice the protein of ordinary yoghurt.
- 500 ml ready-to-drink milkshake – opt for a shake that contains around 20 g protein for convenient refuelling after exercise. Alternatively, make your own speedy version by mixing 3 tsp of milkshake powder with 500 ml of milk.
- 2 × 100 ml yoghurt drinks plus 300 ml milk-based drink. Probiotic yoghurt drinks are useful for boosting immunity, thanks to their probiotic bacteria, as well as supplying protein (3 g), carbohydrate (12 g) and calcium.
- 80 g 'protein' bar. Bars containing a mixture of carbohydrate and whey protein are a convenient option after workouts. Opt for one containing around 20 g protein.

if your maintenance calorie requirement is 2700 kcal, you will need to eat 2700 x 1.2 = 3240 kcal.

Here are nine top tips for weight gain:

- Put more total eating time into your daily routine. This may mean rescheduling other activities. Plan your meal and snack times in advance and never skip or rush them, no matter how busy you are.
- Increase your meal frequency – eat at least three meals and three snacks daily.
- Get into the habit of eating every 3–4 hours. Going 5 or more hours between meals makes

Monitor your body composition

Measuring your body fat percentage using skinfold calipers or bioelectrical impedance will tell you how much of you is muscle and how much of you is fat (see page 53). In gaining weight, expect some of that to be fat. If you put on 3 kg of muscle and 1 kg of fat, you're making great progress. If you gained 2 kg of muscle and 2 kg of fat over the same period, you know your overall calorie and carbohydrate intake is too high, pushing up body fat levels.

If you're not gaining weight...
– Eat one and a half times the amount of carbs and protein at two of your meals a day. Use extra fats (butter, olive oil or coconut oil) and follow the rules on this page.

If you're gaining weight, but it's as much fat as it is muscle...
– Halve the carbs in your meals (excluding your post-workout meal).

If you gained muscle at first, but now your body fat has increased...
– Halve your carbs in your last two meals. If your body fat falls in 2 weeks, increase your carbs.

High-calorie snacks for hard gainers

- Nuts
- Dried fruit
- Milkshake
- Smoothie
- Whole milk or Greek yoghurt
- Yoghurt drink
- Sandwich, bagel, roll, pitta
- Granola or oat-based bar
- Flapjack
- Meal replacement or protein shake
- Protein bar

you more likely to store fat, burn muscle and promote fluctuating blood sugar levels, leaving you tired and weak.
- Plan nutritious high-calorie snacks – e.g. shakes, smoothies, yoghurt, nuts, dried fruit, energy/protein bars.

- Eat larger meals and increase portion sizes – but avoid overfilling!
- If you are finding it hard to eat enough food, try nutrient-dense drinks such as whole milk, flavoured milk, milkshakes, and yoghurt and fruit smoothies to help increase your calorie and protein intake.
- Use whole milk instead of skimmed; strained Greek yoghurt or whole milk yoghurt instead of low-fat varieties.
- Use a little more olive (or rapeseed or coconut) oil for cooking, drizzle olive or walnut oil on salads and veg; scatter extra grated cheese on dishes; add extra butter to toast, sandwiches and sauces.
- Add extra nuts, dried fruit and honey to porridge; stir nuts and honey (or maple syrup) into Greek or whole milk yoghurt.

BUILD MUSCLE NOT FAT

EATING FOR WEIGHT LOSS

Numerous studies have found that the most effective way to lose body fat is by combining regular exercise (ideally both resistance training and cardiovascular exercise) with a modest and sustainable calorie reduction.

Long-term weight control is about making simple yet lasting changes to the way you eat. Your eating plan should include all food groups – in particular foods that satisfy your appetite, foods containing low-glycaemic carbohydrates, and foods with a high content of fibre and water. Here are eight simple ways to shed fat without sacrificing hard-earned muscle.

1. Don't diet

Many popular diets are based on gimmicks or unproven science and often involve cutting out certain food categories or limiting carbohydrates. They may help you lose weight in the short term but the problem is that they are not sustainable. Sooner or later, you'll end up eating the banned foods, giving up the diet and putting the weight back on.

2. Eat 'real' food

Losing fat is far easier if you focus on basic or 'real' foods, i.e. minimally processed foods that resemble something you may find in nature. These foods are more filling and satiating than processed foods, which automatically limits the amount of calories you consume without needing much restraint.

3. Adjust carbs

The key to fat loss is to adjust your carbohydrate intake. This doesn't mean forgoing pasta or potatoes, but reducing it to a level that gives you just enough fuel for your training but not too little to cause fatigue or illness. Training at high intensities with low glycogen levels will eventually result in fatigue and poor performance. You'll need to eat less than your 'maintenance' level and you'll need to eat more on days when your energy needs are higher (i.e. on training days). For most people, this is likely to average 3–5 g carbohydrate/kg body weight/day.

4. Don't be afraid of fat

Fat is high in calories so reducing the amount of fat you eat is a good way of lowering the calorie density of your diet. However, don't cut it out completely; fat is also satiating, so it gives the body the feeling of being full – providing you eat it in as natural a form as possible (e.g. milk, cheese, nuts, avocado, oily fish). Avoid anything labeled 'low fat', 'reduced fat' or 'fat free' – they are often higher in sugar and calories than the full-fat versions to make up for the flavour and texture that's lost when food manufacturers take out the fat.

Fats should still provide around 20–35 per cent of your calories, with a balance of saturated and unsaturated fats. Cut down heavily processed foods that combine fats and carbohydrates (crisps, pastries, pies, biscuits, desserts and cakes) as they are not only high in calories but also provide poor satiety and may make you overeat.

5. Keep protein in the mix

High-protein foods suppress the appetite longer and help prolong satiety more than foods high in carbohydrate or fat, which is why it is particularly useful when you're trying to shed fat. In fact, slightly upping your protein intake may help maintain your muscle mass while dieting. One study found that when athletes ate 1.6 g or 2.4 g protein/kg body weight (2 or 3 times the RDA), they lost more fat and less muscle compared with those who just ate the RDA for protein, 0.8 g/kg body weight (Pasiakos *et al*, 2013). Include 2–4 portions (140–280 g total weight) of high-protein foods (poultry, fish, dairy foods, beans, eggs, tofu) daily. But remember, eating more protein than you need won't help you lose weight faster, boost metabolism or build muscle!

6. Choose naturally fibre-rich foods

Eating more fibre-rich foods, such as fruit, vegetables, beans and whole grains, can help satisfy hunger and reduce calorie intake. Fibre expands in the gut, making you feel full, and so helps to stop you overeating. It helps to satisfy your hunger by slowing the rate that foods pass through your digestive system and stabilising blood sugar levels. Also, fibre-rich foods require more chewing, which helps slow down your eating and prevents you overeating. Eating slowly gives your brain the chance to recognise that you're full.

7. Add cardiovascular exercise

Cardiovascular exercise burns calories and increases the body's ability to burn fat. It includes any kind of activity that uses the large muscle groups of the body and can be kept up for 20–40 minutes, with your heart rate in your target training range (60–85 per cent of maximum heart rate). Try running, elliptical training machines, swimming, cycling, fast walking and group exercise classes. Vary your activities so you don't become bored. Remember, the higher the resistance, the more muscle you will build, so high-resistance activities such as rowing, stair-climbing, incline running and hard cycling are good for strengthening as well

as defining muscles. The ACSM recommends 150 minutes per week to improve cardiovascular health (Garber *et al*, 2011) or 200–300 minutes to lose weight. This can be met through 30–60 minutes of moderate-intensity exercise (5 days per week) or 20–60 minutes of vigorous-intensity exercise (3 days per week). Increase the intensity and duration of your sessions gradually, aiming for 60 minutes 5 times a week.

But don't overdo it. Studies have shown that after about 60–90 minutes of aerobic activity, the body begins to break down and use muscle tissue as fuel and, on a calorie-restricted diet, this happens earlier on in your workout. Your basic metabolic rate slows, so you won't burn as many calories.

8. Keep a food diary

Keeping a food diary will give you a much clearer idea of where your calories are coming from. Use a calorie counter app such as myfitnesspal or a simple pad and pen to keep a daily food diary. Identify the foods or drinks that aren't helping your fat loss efforts. Work out which types of food you need to reduce or increase. Main culprits are likely to be calorie-dense low-fibre snacks: biscuits, puddings, crisps, ice cream, cakes and chocolate bars.

CORE MENU PLANS FOR MUSCLE GAIN

Here are three core menu plans, providing different amounts of energy, designed to help you gain muscle. They give you the amounts of foods needed to meet your calorie and macronutrient requirements. They provide approximately 3000, 3500 and 4000 calories and are suitable for indviduals weighing less than 65 kg, less than 75 kg and more than 75 kg respectively and doing approximately 1 to 2 hours moderate-intensity training a day. If you exercise longer than an hour a day or at a very high intensity then you should increase the portion sizes to take account of your greater calorie expenditure.

You should use the core menu plans as a template for developing your individual daily eating plan. Where the menu plan gives a choice of food type (e.g. 'carbs'), simply pick your preferred option (e.g. pasta or potatoes) or substitute an equivalent (high carb) food (e.g. quinoa or noodles). Try to vary your choice of fresh fruit and vegetables as much as possible according to what's in season as this will give you a greater range of micronutrients, antioxidants and phytonutrients.

Measure and weigh your portions carefully to start with to get an idea of what different amounts of foods look like. Thereafter, you should find it quicker and easier to judge how much to eat.

You should also track your progress – if you're not gaining muscle, then you may need to increase your portion sizes overall; if you're gaining fat as well as muscle then you may need to reduce the carbs in your meals.

The menu plans do not give quantities for water or other drinks as the amount you need is quite individual and will vary day to day according to the climate and your sweat rate.

The menu plans provide guidance on 'real' foods but do not give recommendations for sports supplements or products. Read the information in Chapter 8 before deciding to incorporate any product into your daily eating plan.

Table 7.7	Core menu plan for muscle gain (for < 65 kg person)
Breakfast	Water 2 eggs plus 2 slices wholegrain toast 300 ml milk (or hot chocolate/coffee/milkshake) 100 g fresh fruit
Snack	25 g nuts 100 g fresh fruit Water
Lunch	*Protein:* 150 g chicken, meat, fish or 3 eggs or 75 g cheese Vegetables or salad *Carbs:* 3 slices wholegrain bread or 75 g (uncooked weight) wholegrain pasta or rice or 300 g potato *Fat:* 15 g olive/coconut oil or butter 100 g fresh fruit and 125 g whole milk yoghurt Water
Pre-training	2 bananas 125 g whole milk yoghurt Water
Training (< 2 h)	100 ml cordial or squash (diluted 1:8)
Post-training	600 ml milk/milkshake/protein shake 125 g whole milk yoghurt
Dinner	Water *Protein:* 150 g meat, chicken or fish or 3 eggs or 75 g cheese Vegetables or salad *Carbs:* 75 g (uncooked weight) wholegrain pasta or rice or 300 g potato *Fat:* 15 g olive/coconut oil or butter 100 g fresh fruit and 125 g whole milk yoghurt *Nutritional analysis:* Calories 3006 198 g protein (26% calories) 101 g fat (30% calories) 351 g carbohydrate (44% calories)

Table 7.8	Core menu plan for muscle gain (for < 75 kg person)
Breakfast	Water Porridge (75 g oatmeal plus 500 ml milk) Banana 2 eggs plus 1 slice wholegrain toast
Snack	25 g nuts 100 g fresh fruit Water
Lunch	Water *Protein:* 150 g chicken, meat, fish or 3 eggs or 75 g cheese Vegetables or salad *Carbs:* 3 slices wholegrain bread or 75 g (uncooked weight) wholegrain pasta or rice or 300 g potato *Fat:* 15 g olive/coconut oil or butter 100 g fresh fruit and 125 g whole milk yoghurt
Snack	2 bananas 125 g whole milk yoghurt Water
Training (< 2 h)	100 ml cordial or squash (diluted 1:8)
Snack	600 ml milk/protein shake 125 g whole milk yoghurt
Dinner	Water *Protein:* 150 g chicken, meat or fish or 3 eggs or 75 g cheese Vegetables or salad *Carbs:* 75 g (uncooked weight) wholegrain pasta or rice or 300 g potato *Fat:* 15 g olive/coconut oil or butter 100 g fresh fruit and 125 g whole milk yoghurt
	Nutritional analysis: 3425 calories 212 g protein (25% calories) 111 g fat (29% calories) 425 g carbohydrate (46% calories)

Table 7.9	Core menu plan for muscle gain (for > 75 kg person)
Breakfast	Water Porridge (75 g oatmeal plus 500 ml milk) Banana 2 eggs plus 2 slices wholegrain toast
Snack	50 g nuts 100 g fresh fruit Water
Lunch	Water *Protein:* 150 g chicken, meat, fish or 3 eggs or 75 g cheese Vegetables or salad *Carbs:* 4 slices bread or 100 g wholegrain pasta or rice or 400 g potato *Fat:* 25 g olive/coconut oil or butter 100 g fresh fruit and 125 g whole milk yoghurt
Snack	2 bananas 125 g whole milk yoghurt Water
Training (< 2 h)	100 ml cordial or squash (diluted 1:8)
Snack	600 ml milk/protein shake 125 g whole milk yoghurt
Dinner	Water *Protein:* 150 g chicken, meat or fish or 3 eggs or 75 g cheese Vegetables or salad *Carbs:* 75 g (uncooked weight) wholegrain pasta or rice or 300 g potato *Fat:* 25 g olive/coconut oil or butter 100 g fresh fruit and 125 g whole milk yoghurt *Nutritional analysis:* 4010 calories 226 g protein (22% calories) 147 g fat (33% calories) 480 g carbohydrate (45% calories)

SUMMARY OF KEY POINTS

- To gain weight, you need to take in more calories (approximately 20 per cent) than you burn.
- To reduce body fat and maintain muscle, reduce calories by no more than 15 per cent.
- The general guideline for carbohydrate intake is 5–7 g/kg body weight/day.
- Hypertrophy occurs when you are in positive protein balance, i.e. MPS exceeds muscle protein breakdown.
- For building and maintaining muscle mass, it is recommended that strength trainers consume 1.6–1.8 g protein/kg body weight/day, and up to 2.4 g/kg body weight during calorie restriction (dieting).
- Consuming protein in the immediate post-training period increases muscle protein synthesis MPS; however, the post-anabolic window lasts for up to 24 hours.
- The ideal post-workout intake is 20–25 g protein or 0.25–0.3 g/kg body weight. This amount should also be included in each meal to promote optimal protein synthesis.
- High-quality proteins, such as milk and whey, are particularly beneficial for MPS as they are rapidly digested as well as being rich in leucine and other EAAs.
- There is no specific recommendation for fat – it provides the balance of calories after subtracting your carbohydrate and protein requirement.
- Eating a low-GI meal 2–4 hours before training can help maintain blood sugar levels during your workout.
- Carbohydrate plus protein, in a ratio of approximately 3:1, promotes the fastest post-exercise recovery of glycogen and creates a more favourable anabolic environment for muscle growth.

SPORTS SUPPLEMENTS

8

With the ever-growing number of supplements available online, in supermarkets, health stores and gyms, it is tempting to think that all those shakes, powders and pills will give you the edge when it comes to building muscle or improving performance. The simple truth is that they will not. Proper nutrition in combination with a consistent strength-training programme and adequate rest is far more important than supplementation when it comes to optimising performance. Taking supplements cannot compensate for a poorly planned diet, inconsistent training or lack of rest. Only once these fundamental pillars are in place should you consider supplementation.

It is important to know that there is no systematic regulation of supplements. This means that there is no guarantee that the product contains what is stated on the label or lives up to its claims. Worse, there is a risk that uncertified products could be contaminated with banned substances. This is known to be the case as many athletes have been tested positive through the use of such supplements. An investigation by the Medicines and Healthcare Products Regulatory Agency found illegal substances, such as steroids, stimulants and hormones, in 84 sports supplements in the UK (MHRA, 2012).

A survey by HFL Sport Science found 10 per cent of a sample of 114 of the most popular supplements and weight loss products purchased in Europe were contaminated with steroids and/ or stimulants (Russell *et al*, 2013). Some of the contaminated products even claimed to have been 'tested by an independent laboratory' or that they were 'doping free'.

The World Anti-Doping Code contains the principle of 'strict liability'. That means that the athlete is strictly liable for any prohibited substances found in their bodies. Should you decide to take a supplement, you can minimise the risk of inadvertent doping by looking for voluntary certifications by companies such as Informed-Sport or NSF Certified for Sport (US) on the label. This indicates that the product has been independently tested for banned substances. You'll find all registered products listed on the companies' websites www.informed-sport.com and www.nsfsport.com.

If you are considering taking supplements, you need to know whether they are effective, safe and legal. The majority of supplements marketed to athletes are little more than hype – only a small handful are supported by strong evidence. Here is an evaluation of the science behind the most popular sports supplements to help you make a properly informed decision.

ANTIOXIDANTS

What are they?
Antioxidant supplements include beta-carotene, vitamin C, vitamin E, zinc, magnesium, copper, lycopene (a pigment found in tomatoes), selenium, co-enzyme Q10, catechins (found in green tea), methionine (an amino acid) and anthocyanidins (pigments found in purple or red fruit).

How do they work?
The theory behind antioxidant supplementation is that it may reduce the damage caused by free radicals (reactive oxygen species, ROS) during intense exercise and speed recovery.

What is the evidence?
Studies suggest that exercise itself increases the oxidative capacity of muscles by enhancing the action of the body's own antioxidant enzymes such as glutathione peroxidase and superoxide dismutase (Draeger *et al*, 2014). In other words, the body adapts to exercise by increasing its own antioxidant defences. Thus, taking supplements will provide no further benefit.

In fact, studies have found that supplements may delay rather than promote recovery after exercise (Nikolaidis *et al*, 2012). One double-blind randomised controlled trial found that taking vitamin C (1000 mg) and E (235 mg) after exercise hampered adaptations in the muscle cells and provided no performance benefit (Paulsen *et al*, 2013). A review of more than 150 studies concluded that high doses of antioxidant supplements do not improve performance (Peternelj & Coombes, 2011).

It is thought that oxidative stress (caused by ROS) is desirable as it helps stimulate muscle growth and recovery. Thus, taking high doses of supplements to quench these ROS prevents muscle adaptations.

Are there any side effects?
Antioxidant supplementation may delay recovery and reduce performance.

Verdict
There is no benefit to be gained from taking high dose antioxidant supplements. Instead of improving performance or promoting recovery, supplements may actually hamper it by disrupting the mechanisms designed to deal with exercise-derived oxidative stress. The consensus statement by the ACSM cautions against the use of antioxidant supplements (Rodriguez *et al*, 2009).

Getting your vitamins and minerals through a varied and balanced diet remains the best approach to maintain an optimal antioxidant status. There's good evidence to suggest that a diet rich in foods that are naturally high in antioxidants is associated with better health outcomes.

BEETROOT JUICE

What is it?
Beetroot juice (and, of course, beetroot) is a rich source of nitrate. Nitrate is also found in other vegetables, such as spinach, rocket, celeriac, cabbage, endive, leeks and broccoli.

How does it work?
The nitrates in beetroot juice are converted in the body into nitric oxide (NO), a potent vasodilator

(widens blood vessels) that helps increase blood flow and delivery of oxygen and nutrients to the muscles, thereby lowering the amount of oxygen needed by exercising muscles to sustain sub-maximal exercise.

What is the evidence?

Since 2009, a number of studies with non-elite athletes have shown that nitrate in the form of beetroot juice may help sustain higher levels of power for longer before fatigue sets in. In summary, it appears to reduce maximal oxygen uptake, improve exercise economy so you need less energy to do the same amount of work, and allow you to exercise longer.

A review of 17 studies by UK and Australian researchers concluded that nitrate in the form of either beetroot juice or sodium nitrate significantly improved endurance, as measured by time to exhaustion (Hoon *et al*, 2013).

It's important to note that the majority of studies showing a positive effect involved untrained or recreational athletes, not elite athletes. Whether beetroot juice also benefits performance in elite athletes is unclear. For example, Australian researchers found that beetroot juice supplementation (with or without caffeine) did not improve performance in competitive cyclists (Lane *et al*, 2013). Another study with competitive cyclists found little difference in time trial performance following beetroot juice supplementation (Hoon *et al*, 2014).

Are there any side effects?

Beetroot juice may cause a harmless, temporary, pink coloration of urine and stools. It may also trigger 'digestive distress'.

Verdict

If you're a non-elite athlete, beetroot juice may help to give you the edge during endurance exercise lasting between 4 and 30 minutes, or during intense intermittent exercise and team sports. Whether the same benefits apply to the elite athlete is not known for certain. Most studies have shown benefits with 0.3–0.4 g (0.62 mg/kg body weight), equivalent to 500 ml beetroot juice or 170 ml beetroot juice concentrate or a single 70 ml concentrated 'shot' or 200 g cooked beetroot (equivalent to 300 mg nitrate).

However, 600 mg nitrate may be optimal, equivalent to 2 x 70 ml concentrated beetroot shots, taken 2½ hours pre-exercise (Wylie *et al*, 2013). You should avoid using antibacterial mouthwash as this removes the beneficial bacteria in the mouth that convert some of the nitrate to nitrite and thus reduces the benefits of beetroot juice.

BETA-ALANINE

What is it?

Beta-alanine is an amino acid that is used to make carnosine (a dipeptide made from beta-alanine and histidine). Carnosine is an important pH buffer in the muscles that reduces the acidity produced during high-intensity exercise.

How does it work?

Beta-alanine supplementation increases carnosine concentration in the muscle (Harris *et al*, 2006; Sale *et al*, 2010), which increases its buffering capacity, reduces the build-up of lactic acid during high-intensity exercise and delays fatigue.

What is the evidence?

A systematic review of 19 randomised controlled studies concluded that beta-alanine supplementation leads to improved performance in short-duration high-intensity activities (Quesnele *et al*, 2014). It appears to work by increasing power output and anaerobic capacity, and decreasing subjective feelings of fatigue and perceived exhaustion. According to an analysis of 15 studies, the average performance improvement is 2.85 per cent, equivalent to a 6-second improvement in an event lasting 4 minutes (Hobson *et al*, 2012).

Are there any side effects?

High doses may cause side effects such as flushing and paraesthesia (skin tingling). However, these symptoms are normally transient and can be prevented by using smaller doses or sustained-release formulations. The long-term effects of supplements are not known.

Verdict

Beta-alanine supplementation could be beneficial for strength training as it improves performance in activities that last between 1 and 4 minutes or involve repeated sprints or surges of power. However, the research to date has involved relatively small numbers of athletes, so opinions may change as further research is carried out. The optimal dose appears to be around 3 g (4 x 800 mg) per day for 6 weeks followed by a maintenance dose of 1.2 g/day.

BRANCHED CHAIN AMINO ACIDS

What are they?

Branched chain amino acids consist of the three amino acids that have a branched molecular configuration: valine, leucine and isoleucine. Muscles may use BCAAs for fuel when muscle glycogen is depleted.

How do they work?

The theory behind supplementation is that BCAA can help prevent the breakdown of muscle tissue during intense exercise.

What is the evidence?

Some data show that BCAA supplementation before and after exercise may decrease exercise-induced muscle damage and promote muscle-protein synthesis (Shimomura *et al*, 2010; Jackman *et al*, 2010; MacLean *et al*, 1994). There is also some evidence that BCAA supplements may help preserve muscle in athletes who are dieting and, taken before resistance training, reduce delayed onset muscle soreness (Nosaka *et al*, 2006). On the other hand, if sufficient protein is being consumed then there appears to be little benefit in taking BCAA supplements.

Are there any side effects?

BCAAs are relatively safe because they are normally found in protein in the diet. Excessive intake may reduce the absorption of other amino acids.

Verdict

BCAAs are found in good amounts in most protein foods and supplements (especially whey protein supplements) and meal replacement products, so it is probably not worth taking them if you already use one of these products. Theoretically, if you aren't getting sufficient protein in your diet or you're not consuming many food sources of BCAAs (e.g. dairy products), then supplements may help reduce muscle protein breakdown and promote muscle synthesis. However, it would make more sense to consume sufficient high-quality protein from food sources (1.2–1.8 g/kg) than rely on supplements to get your amino acids, even if you are dieting.

CAFFEINE

What is it?

Caffeine is a drug rather than a nutrient. However, it is often considered a dietary supplement because it is found in many everyday foods and drinks such as coffee, black and green tea, cola, chocolate, energy drinks and gels.

How does it work?

Caffeine is a stimulant that acts on the central and peripheral nervous system. It works by increasing levels of ß-endorphins (hormone-like substances) in the brain. These endorphins affect mood state, reduce the perception of fatigue and pain, and create a sense of well-being. Thus caffeine helps increase alertness, concentration and performance, and reduce fatigue. It can also help increase fibre recruitment and thereby boost performance in anaerobic activities.

What is the evidence?

Studies suggest that caffeine enhances performance in sprints, high-intensity activities lasting 4–5 minutes, intermittent activities such as team sports, and endurance activities (Burke, 2008; Goldstein et al, 2010).

An analysis by UK researchers of 40 studies on caffeine and performance concluded that it significantly improves endurance, on average by 12 per cent (Doherty & Smith, 2004). A study at the University of Saskatchewan found that consuming caffeine in amounts equivalent to 2 mg caffeine/kg body weight 1 hour before exercise significantly increased bench press muscle endurance (Forbes et al, 2007). Another study, with footballers, found that consuming a caffeinated drink 1 hour before training and then at 15-minute intervals improved sprinting performance and reduced the perception of fatigue (Gant et al, 2010). Caffeine also appears to benefit performance in team sports. Women soccer players who consumed 3 mg caffeine/kg body weight in the form of an energy drink were able to run further and faster in a simulated match (Lara et al, 2014).

Are there any side effects?

Some people may experience side effects such as tremors, increased heart rate and headaches. Other side effects caused by taking too large a dose include nausea, irritability, diarrhoea, insomnia, trembling and nervousness.

Verdict

Caffeine appears to be an effective ergogenic aid, enhancing performance for most types of endurance, power and strength activities. It delays fatigue, reduces perceived effort and increases mental sharpness. It was once classed as a banned substance but is currently legal in most drug-tested competitions.

The optimal dose is 1–3 mg/kg body weight taken approximately 30–60 minutes before exercise. This is equivalent to 70–210 mg (1–2 cups of coffee) for a 70 kg person. Alternatively, you can take caffeine during a workout (if you are exercising longer than an hour) or during the latter stages as fatigue begins to occur. Caffeine pills or 'shots' may give you a more precise dose than coffee or tea as caffeine levels vary considerably so it's hard to know how much you are getting.

CREATINE

What is it?
Creatine is a protein that is made naturally in the body from three amino acids (arginine, glycine and methionine), but is also found in meat and fish.

How does it work?
Creatine supplements increase muscle stores of phosphocreatine (PC). This is an energy-rich compound that is used to re-synthesise ATP and thus fuel muscles during high-intensity activities, such as lifting weights or sprinting. Boosting PC levels with supplements should enable you to sustain all-out effort longer than usual and recover faster between exertions or exercise 'sets', resulting in greater strength and improved ability to do repeated sets.

Creatine may also buffer excess hydrogen ions during high-intensity exercise, allowing more lactic acid to be produced before fatigue sets in. It also helps promote muscle growth by drawing water into the cells, which increases muscle cell volume and acts as a signal for protein synthesis.

What is the evidence?
There is a large amount of research supporting the benefits of creatine supplementation for increasing strength and muscle mass as well as enhancing performance in high-intensity activities (Gualano *et al*, 2012).

A review of 22 studies concluded that creatine supplementation increases maximum strength (i.e. 1 rep maximum) by an average 8 per cent as well as endurance strength, i.e. maximum reps at a sub-maximal load, by 14 per cent (Cooper *et al*, 2012; Rawson & Volek, 2003). Creatine supplementation results in lean mass and total mass gains of typically 1–3 per cent lean body weight (approx. 0.8–3 kg) after a 5-day loading dose, compared with controls (Buford *et al*, 2007).

Are there any side effects?
The main side effect is weight gain. This is due partly to extra water in the muscle cells and partly to increased muscle tissue. While this is desirable for most people, it could be disadvantageous in sports where there is a critical ratio of body weight to speed (e.g. for runners) or in weight-category sports.

Verdict
If you train with weights, or do any sport that includes repeated bursts of high-intensity effort, such as sprints, jumps or throws, then taking creatine supplements may help increase your power, strength, muscle mass and performance.

You may take creatine either as a 'loading protocol' – 20 g for 5–7 days (as 4 x 5 g) – or as smaller doses (2–3 g/day) for 3–4 weeks to achieve optimal levels in your muscles. The end result is the same, whichever method you use. Creatine stores can be maintained by taking 2 g/day (0.03 g/kg body weight). It may be beneficial to take creatine immediately after your workout (Cribb & Hayes, 2006). Opt for creatine monohydrate

– this is the form used in the majority of studies. Other forms, such as citrate, phosphate, malate, pyruvate and serum, are more expensive and less effective.

FAT BURNERS AND STIMULANTS

What are they?
Fat burners include ephedrine, yohimbine, methylhexaneamine (DMAA); citrus aurantium (synephrine or bitter orange extract); green tea extract and *Coleus forskohlii* extract (a herb, similar to mint). Ephedrine is a stimulant substance derived from the ephedra or má huáng plant.

How do they work?
Fat burners and stimulants claim to speed your metabolism, increase alertness, and shed body fat.

What is the evidence?
There is some evidence that ephedrine increases weight loss: partly due to an increase in thermogenesis (heat production), and partly due to its effect on appetite suppression (Coffey *et al*, 2004). In one study, volunteers who took a combination of caffeine and ephedrine before sprinting achieved a better performance than those who took caffeine only, ephedrine only or a placebo (Bell, 2001).

However, there is no sound scientific evidence to back up the weight loss claims of the other ingredients in fat burners. Green tea may stimulate thermogenesis, increasing calorie expenditure, fat burning and weight loss (Dulloo *et al*, 1999).

Are there any side effects?
Ephedrine, yohimbine, synephrine and DMAA can cause significant side effects, such as increased and irregular heartbeat, raised blood pressure, kidney failure and seizures. More severe consequences such as heart attack, stroke and death have been reported in the press. Several athletes have tested positive for DMAA and it has been linked to a number of fatalities. Citrus aurantium can increase blood pressure as much, if not more, than ephedrine. High doses of forskolin may cause heart disturbances.

Verdict
Ephedrine, yohimbine, synephrine and methylhexaneamine (DMAA) are banned substances prohibited by WADA in drug-tested competitions (WADA, 2014). The research on ephedrine-free fat burners is not robust and any fat-burning boost they provide would be relatively small or none.

GLUTAMINE

What is it?
Glutamine is a non-essential amino acid found abundantly in the muscle cells and blood. It is found in high-protein foods, such as meat, fish, milk and eggs.

What does it do?
Glutamine is needed for cell growth as well as serving as a fuel for the immune system. Supplementation during intense training periods is thought to reduce the exercise-induced drop in glutamine, boost immunity, reduce the risk of overtraining syndrome and prevent upper respiratory tract infections. It has also been suggested that glutamine may have a protein-sparing effect during intense training.

What is the evidence?

A review of studies concluded that while many athletes take glutamine supplements to protect against exercise-related impairment of the immune system, supplements do not prevent post-exercise changes in immune function or reduce the risk of infection (Gleeson, 2008).

One study found that there was no difference in plasma glutamine concentrations between elite swimmers who developed upper respiratory tract infections (URTI) and those who didn't during a 4-week period of intense training, suggesting that URTI is not related to changes in plasma glutamine concentration (Mackinnon & Hooper, 1996).

To date, few studies have looked at the effects of glutamine supplements on sports performance. A review of studies concluded that there is little scientific evidence that glutamine can improve muscle mass, reduce body fat or improve performance (Phillips, 2007).

Are there any side effects?

No side effects have been identified.

Verdict

There is little evidence to support the benefits of glutamine supplementation. It is unlikely to increase immunity or improve muscle mass, strength or sports performance.

HMB (BETA-HYDROXY BETA-METHYLBUTYRATE)

What is it?

HMB is a metabolite of the BCAA leucine. Your body breaks down leucine into HMB, but you can also get it from grapefruit, catfish and alfalfa.

How does it work?

HMB is a precursor to a component of cell membranes, which helps with the growth and repair of muscle tissue. Its role is not yet clear but scientists believe it either helps protect the muscle from excessive breakdown during intense exercise or accelerates muscle repair after training.

What is the evidence?

The evidence for HMB is divided. A number of studies suggest that HMB may have anti-catabolic effects, reducing muscle breakdown after resistance exercise, while others have found no beneficial effect.

A review of studies published by the International Society of Sports Nutrition concluded that HMB promotes recovery, reduces exercise-induced muscle breakdown and damage, promotes muscle repair, and increases muscle mass (Wilson *et al*, 2013).

But these benefits have not been found in all studies, particularly those involving more experienced athletes (Kreider *et al*, 2000). New Zealand researchers found that HMB supplements produced a small increase in strength in novice gym goers but not in more experienced lifters (Rowlands & Thomson, 2009). One Australian study found that 6 weeks of HMB supplementation had no effect on the strength or muscle mass gains of well-conditioned athletes (Slater *et al*, 2001). Researchers at the University of Queensland in

Australia found no beneficial effect on reducing muscle damage or muscle soreness following resistance exercise (Paddon-Jones *et al*, 2001).

Are there any side effects?
No side effects have yet been found.

Verdict

HMB may provide muscle-building benefits for those who are new to lifting weights, but gains are likely to be fairly small compared with other dietary measures you can take. These include consuming enough calories (you should be in a slight positive calorie balance), carbohydrate, protein and fat. Establishing a good nutritional base and a consistent training programme should be your priority before considering supplementation with HMB. Studies have used doses of 1–2 g free acid form HMB 30–60 minutes prior to exercise (or 60–120 minutes prior to exercise if consuming calcium HMB) or 3 g (divided into 3 x 1 g doses)/day for 2 weeks. But HMB is unlikely to be useful for more experienced athletes.

LEUCINE

What is it?
Leucine is an essential amino acid, which means the body cannot produce it and we must get it from dietary sources. Leucine is the most abundant of the three branched chain amino acids (BCAAs) in muscles (the other two are isoleucine and valine).

How does it work?
Leucine is an important trigger for protein synthesis. It acts as a signal to the muscle cells to make new muscle proteins, activating a compound called mTOR (Mammalian Target of Rapamycin), and a molecular switch that turns on the machinery that manufactures muscle proteins.

What is the evidence?
Research suggests that leucine can stimulate protein synthesis (when consumed after exercise) and lessen protein breakdown (when consumed before exercise). In a study at the University of Maastricht, athletes who consumed a leucine/carbohydrate/protein drink after resistance training had less muscle protein breakdown and greater muscle protein synthesis than those who consumed a supplement without leucine (Koopman *et al*, 2005). Similarly, another study found that consuming a leucine-enriched protein drink during endurance exercise resulted in less muscle breakdown and greater muscle synthesis (Pasiakos *et al*, 2011). However, there is no benefit to taking extra leucine if you consume protein (as food or drink) before or after exercise. Researchers found that consuming more than 1.8 g leucine does not produce any additional benefit (Pasiakos & McClung, 2011).

Are there any side effects?
There are no reported side effects.

Verdict

Getting sufficient leucine is particularly important for those wanting to build strength and muscle mass. However, it isn't necessary to get leucine in the form of supplements. It is found widely in foods, the best sources being eggs, dairy products, meat, fish and poultry. It is also found in high concentrations in whey protein. You'll need around 2 g leucine to get maximum muscle-building benefits; that's the amount found in

SPORTS SUPPLEMENTS

approximately 20 g of an animal protein source. Table 8.1 shows the amounts of various foods that you would need to consume to get 2 g leucine and 20 g protein.

Table 8.1	Foods supplying 2 g leucine and 20 g protein
Food	**Amount**
Milk	600 ml
Cheddar cheese	85 g
Plain yoghurt	450 g
Eggs	3
Meat or poultry	85 g
Fish	100 g
Whey powder	17 g

MULTIVITAMINS

What are they?
Multivitamin and mineral supplements contain a mixture of micronutrients.

How do they work?
Regular intense exercise places additional demands on your body, which means the requirement for many micronutrients is likely to be higher than the RDAs for the general population. Micronutrients play an important role in energy production, haemoglobin synthesis, bone health, immune function and protection of the body against oxidative damage. They help with synthesis and repair of muscle tissue during recovery. As a result, greater intakes of micronutrients may be required to cover increased needs for building, repair and maintenance of lean body mass in athletes. Failure to get enough micronutrients could leave you lacking in energy and susceptible to minor infections and illnesses.

What is the evidence?
Scientific evidence to support the use of multi-vitamins is lacking. Although supplementation may improve the nutritional status of an individual who consumes marginal amounts of nutrients and may enhance the physical performance of those athletes with overt nutrient deficiencies, there is no scientific evidence to support the general use of vitamin and mineral supplements to improve athletic performance. According to the ACSM, the increased food intake of physically active individuals should provide the additional vitamins and minerals needed if a wide variety of foods is included in the diet (Rodriguez *et al*, 2009).

A comprehensive review of 26 studies concluded that for healthy people without nutritional deficiencies, there's little justification for taking multivitamins (Fortmann *et al*, 2013).

Are there any side effects?
Taking multivitamin supplements is generally harmless as amounts of nutrients are usually close to the RDAs. But you should check that they are all within safe upper levels. While you would have to really overdo your vitamin and mineral intake to create serious toxicity issues, even moderate levels of 'mega dosing' can have adverse effects.

Verdict
If you are consuming a healthy diet that meets your calorie and macronutrient requirements, you probably won't benefit from multivitamin supplements. High doses will not enhance exercise performance or health. On the other hand, supplements providing approximately the

RDA for most nutrients are unlikely to do any harm and may be regarded as useful insurance against deficient intakes.

PROHORMONES

What are they?
Prohormone supplements include DHEA, androstenedione (or andro for short) and nor-androstenedione.

How do they work?
Manufacturers claim the supplements will increase testosterone levels in the body and produce similar muscle-building effects to anabolic steroids, but without the side effects.

What is the evidence?
There is little evidence behind these supplements. Contrary to manufacturers' claims, 'andro' supplements and DHEA fail to raise testosterone or increase muscle mass or strength (Brown *et al*, 1999; King *et al*, 1999; Broeder *et al*, 2000; Powers, 2002).

In a double-blind crossover study, researchers from McMaster University, Canada, found that androstenedione supplements failed to raise testosterone levels in the blood either at rest or following resistance training compared with a placebo (Ballantyne *et al*, 2000).

A study at Iowa State University found that 8 weeks of supplementation with androstenedione, DHEA, saw palmetto, Tribulus terrestris and chrysin combined with a resistance training programme failed to raise testosterone levels or increase muscle strength or mass – in spite of increased levels of androstenedione – compared with a placebo (Brown *et al*, 2000).

Are there any side effects?
Studies have found that prohormones increase oestrogen, which can lead to gynecomastia (male breast development) and decrease HDL (high density lipoprotein) levels (King *et al*, 1999). Reduced HDL carries a greater heart disease risk. Other side effects include acne, enlarged prostate and water retention. Some supplements include anti-oestrogen substances, such as chrysin (dihydroxyflavone), to counteract the side effects, but there is no evidence that they work either (Brown *et al*, 2000).

Verdict
Prohormones are banned substances with no proven benefits. They will not boost testosterone or build muscle, so should be avoided.

RECOVERY DRINKS

What's in them?
Recovery drinks contain a mixture of carbohydrate and protein. The carbohydrate usually comprises sugar and maltodextrin, and the protein may be whey or a mixture of whey, casein and soy.

How do they work?
Consuming protein with carbohydrate stimulates muscle protein synthesis (i.e. muscle repair and growth) and glycogen replenishment, and therefore speeds recovery to a greater extent than carbohydrate or protein alone.

What is the evidence?
Research has shown that consuming a drink containing a 3 to 1 or 4 to 1 ratio of carbohydrate to protein promotes glycogen refuelling after exercise (Phillips *et al*, 2007).

Whey is a 'fast-acting' protein which is rapidly digested and absorbed. It also has all the essential amino acids and high levels of the branched chain amino acid leucine, which has been shown to trigger muscle protein synthesis. Studies have shown that whey is superior to casein and soy in promoting muscle repair after resistance exercise (Tang *et al*, 2009; Churchward-Venne *et al*, 2012). However, casein and soy are added to some brands because they are absorbed slower than whey and so provide a 'timed release' of protein to the muscles. The whey delivers quickly while the casein and soy provide a more sustained rise in blood levels of amino acids, extending the window for muscle building. Side effects are unlikely but check the energy (calorie) content per serving. Excessive intakes may result in weight gain if your 24 hour energy intake exceeds your expenditure.

Verdict

Recovery drinks may be useful for maximising muscle repair and glycogen storage, especially if you're planning to exercise again within 24 hours. The ideal level of carbohydrate is 1–1.5 g of carbohydrate/kg body weight (Rodriguez *et al*, 2009), but you should adjust this depending on the intensity and duration of your workout. The optimal amount of protein that promotes muscle building is 15–25 g (Moore *et al*, 2009). Alternatively, you can drink milk (600 ml provides 20 g protein) or make your own recovery drink (see box). Milk helps rehydrate the body more effectively than sports drinks (Desbrow *et al*, 2014; Shirreffs *et al*, 2007).

TESTOSTERONE BOOSTERS

What are they?
These include *Tribulus terrestris* (a flowering plant), horny goat weed (a leafy plant), and zinc. They are marketed as natural alternatives to anabolic steroids.

How do they work?
Manufacturers claim that the phytochemicals in the plants increase testosterone production and therefore increase muscle mass and strength as well as boosting libido.

What is the evidence?
There is no evidence supporting the claims for *Tribulus terrestris* or horny goat weed. A 4-week study of 21 healthy young men failed to find any measurable differences in testosterone levels between those taking a *Tribulus terrestris* supplement and a placebo group (Neychev & Mitev, 2005). Similarly, a study of 22 Australian elite rugby players found no difference in testosterone levels, nor any improvement in strength or body composition after 5 weeks of supplementation with *Tribulus terrestris* compared with a placebo (Rogerson *et al*, 2007). Despite the manufacturers' claims, there have been no studies on horny goat weed and

---

Make your own recovery drink

Combine 600 ml milk and 2 tablespoons (30 g) milkshake powder (add more or less according to the length, intensity and type of exercise). Or blend 500 ml milk, a banana, 100 ml yoghurt and a scoop (25 g) of whey protein powder.

testosterone levels in humans – only studies with rats!

Zinc supplements do not raise testosterone levels unless you have a deficiency, i.e. abnormally low testosterone levels (see 'ZMA' page 98). By correcting the deficiency, you may notice a short-term improvement in strength and muscle mass.

Are there any side effects?
Tribulus supplements are unlikely to produce side effects. However, they are contraindicated for people with breast or prostate cancer.

Verdict
Despite the claims, testosterone boosters do not increase testosterone, improve muscle mass or enhance athletic performance. Although some manufacturers claim *Tribulus terrestris* will not lead to a positive drug test, others have suggested it may increase the urinary testosterone/epitestosterone (T/E) ratio, which may place athletes at risk of a positive drug test. So you should avoid anything containing this supplement if you compete in a drug-tested sport.

WHEY PROTEIN
What is it?
Whey protein is derived from milk (the by-product of cheese production) and provides a balanced source of all nine essential amino acids, including the branched chain amino acids leucine, isoleucine and valine. There are three types of whey supplements:

Whey protein concentrate – produced by ultrafiltration of whey, and generally contains about 80 per cent protein (the remainder being lactose, fat and water).

Whey protein isolate – produced by a variety of membrane filtration or ion-exchange techniques that remove almost all the lactose and fat, and generally contains more than 90 per cent protein.

Whey protein hydrolysates – produced by enzymatic hydrolysis of whey concentrate or whey isolate, which 'pre-digests' the protein by separating peptide bonds, so it is digested and absorbed faster.

How does it work?
Whey is digested quickly and rapidly absorbed in the intestine. It provides high levels of leucine, which is both a key signal molecule for initiation and an important substrate for new protein synthesis.

What is the evidence?
Studies have found that whey supplements may help increase muscle protein synthesis. In one study, those consuming 20 g of whey supplement before and after resistance exercise had greater increases in muscle mass and muscle strength over 10 weeks compared with those consuming a placebo (Willoughby *et al*, 2007). Another study found that when athletes consumed a whey supplement immediately before and after a training session, they could perform more reps and lift heavier weights 24 hours and 48 hours after the workout compared with those taking a placebo (Hoffman *et al*, 2010).

However, in studies where athletes were already consuming adequate amounts of protein in their diet, taking additional protein in the form of supplements before and after their workouts made no difference to muscle synthesis or strength (Weisgarber *et al*, 2012). There is no evidence to suggest that whey supplements produce faster or greater muscle gains than real food sources of whey, such as milk, yoghurt and cheese. Studies to date have compared whey with carbohydrate, casein or soy supplements, and not with real food.

Are there any side effects?
An excessive intake of protein, whether from food or supplements, is not harmful but offers no health or performance advantage. Concerns about excess protein harming the liver and kidneys or causing calcium loss from the bones have been disproved.

Verdict
If you are getting enough protein from food, there's probably little point in taking supplements. You may prefer to drink milk (which contains whey naturally) as studies have shown that it is just as effective in promoting muscle synthesis after resistance training as supplements. Athletes who consumed milk gained more muscle than those consuming soy protein drinks during a 12-week resistance training programme (Hartman *et al*, 2007).

But if you have higher-than-average requirements or you are a vegetarian or vegan, then whey protein may be a convenient way of adding protein to your diet. Supplements may also be a convenient way of getting your protein when you're out and about.

ZMA
What is it?
ZMA (the acronym for zinc and magnesium aspartate) combines zinc, magnesium, vitamin B6 and aspartate.

How does it work?
It is claimed that ZMA can boost testosterone production, increase strength and improve muscle mass and promote recovery after exercise. Zinc is needed for growth, cell reproduction and testosterone production. In theory, a deficiency may reduce the body's anabolic hormone levels and adversely affect muscle mass and strength. Magnesium is used in the production of energy – a deficiency may reduce endurance.

What is the evidence?
Both zinc and magnesium deficiencies can impair performance (Nielsen & Lukaski, 2006). It is feasible that ZMA supplementation corrects underlying zinc and/or magnesium deficiencies, thus 'normalising' various body processes and improving testosterone levels. This is supported by one study, which found ZMA increased testosterone and strength in a group of football players (Brilla & Conte, 2000). However, this was a small study with a high drop-out rate and has not been replicated since.

A more rigorous randomised, double-blind study with 42 experienced weight-trainers found that supplementation with ZMA for 8 weeks failed to increase testosterone levels, strength, muscle mass, anaerobic capacity or muscular endurance compared with a placebo (Wilborn *et el*, 2004).

Are there any side effects?
High levels of zinc – more than 50 mg – can interfere with the absorption of iron and other minerals, leading to iron deficiency. High doses of magnesium can cause diarrhoea and interfere with calcium absorption.

Verdict

ZMA may be beneficial if you are deficient in zinc and magnesium but otherwise, taking supplements probably won't help you gain muscle mass or get stronger. It cannot be recommended for 'boosting testosterone' or improving performance. You can obtain zinc from whole grains, including wholemeal bread, nuts, beans and lentils. Magnesium is found in nuts, whole grains, green leafy vegetables, fruit and milk.

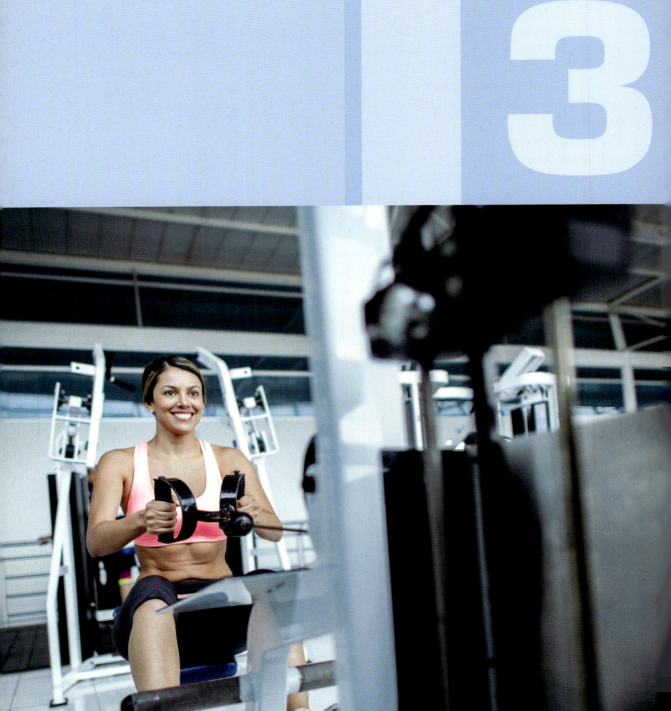

3

PART THREE

THE EXERCISES

In the following chapters, you'll learn how to execute more than 100 exercises with perfect technique. The exercises are divided up by body part: lower body, back, chest, shoulders, arms and abdominals. Each exercise includes step-by-step instructions, technique tips and extra pointers on how to make the exercise harder or easier. There are two photographs demonstrating each exercise, one at the start position and one at the midpoint position. Use these photographs as a guide to correct technique but, in case of doubt, seek the advice of a qualified instructor.

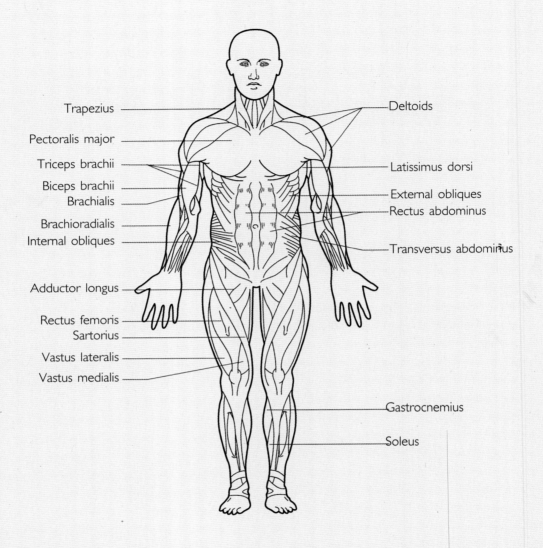

Figure Part 3.1 Muscles of the human body (front view)

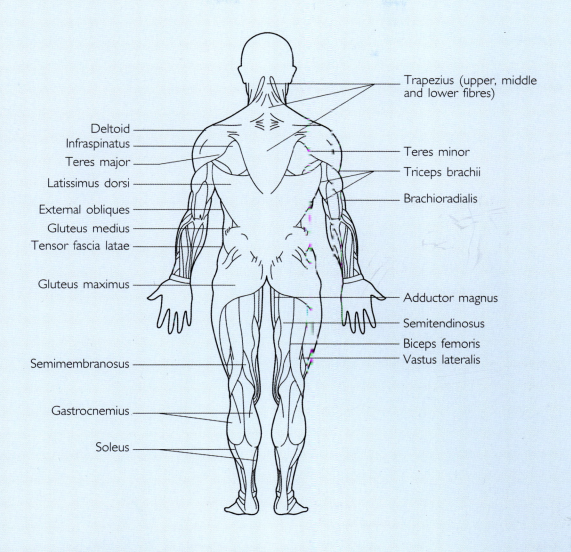

Figure Part 3.2 Muscles of the human body (back view)

// THE LOWER BODY

9

Strong, powerful legs give your body good symmetry, balancing the development of the upper body, and facilitating good performance in other sports.

Building a good foundation of strength in the lower body is important in all sports that require running, jumping, lifting, kicking and pushing. Hip and leg extension plays a major role in:

- running – as seen in athletics, football and rugby
- jumping – as seen in volleyball and netball
- kicking – as seen in football and martial arts.

Lower body exercises not only build strength in the hips and thighs but also stimulate muscle growth in the upper body (Raastad *et al*, 2000). This is because intense leg training (with weights equivalent to 3–6 RM) stimulates the release of anabolic hormones – namely testosterone and growth hormone – which, in turn, improves whole-body muscle growth.

Training the legs with high intensity will also elevate your heart rate and this, together with the resulting muscle mass increase, will allow you to burn fat more efficiently.

EXERCISES FOR THE LOWER BODY

Squat
Front Squat
Split squat
Dead lift
Leg press
Leg extension
Front lunge
Reverse lunge
Walking lunge
Dumbbell step-ups
Seated leg curl
Straight leg dead lift
Standing calf raise
Dumbbell single leg calf raise
Calf (or toe) press

MUSCLE KNOW-HOW

THE LEG MUSCLES

There are four parts (heads) to the muscle at the front of the thigh, known as the quadriceps – the rectus femoris, vastus lateralis, vastus medialis and vastus intermedius – whose collective function is to extend (straighten) the knee. The rectus femoris also flexes the hip – i.e. lifts the thigh up and forwards.

The vastus medialis runs along the inside of the thigh to the rectus femoris and can be seen on the inside of the knee when the leg is locked out; the vastus lateralis runs down the outside of the thigh and can be seen on the outside of the knee; the rectus femoris can be seen when the leg is lifted up and forwards slightly; the vastus intermedius cannot readily be seen as it lies underneath the other muscles.

The main inner-thigh muscles comprise three adductor muscles – adductor brevis, adductor longus and adductor magnus – whose function is to adduct, or pull, the legs together, while the muscles of the outer thigh – the gluteus minimus and gluteus medius – pull the legs out sideways. The muscles at the back of the leg – the hamstrings – include the biceps femoris (long and short heads), semitendinosus and semimembranosus. They have two main actions: to flex (bend) the knee and also extend the hip (pull the thigh backwards).

The calves comprise two muscles: the gastrocnemius and soleus. The gastrocnemius is the larger of the two and lies on top of the soleus. It is worked when the leg is fully straight and has two distinct lobes, which are visible from behind when the calf is flexed. Its role is to straighten the ankle (plantar flexion), to point the toes, and it also helps bend the knee. The soleus is a broad, flat muscle, which is located beneath the gastrocnemius and also helps straighten the

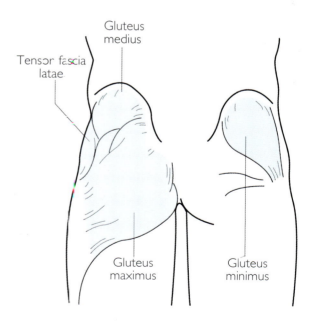

Figure 9.1 Muscles of the leg

Figure 9.2 The gluteal muscles

THE LOWER BODY

105

ankle. It sweeps out to the sides and over across the shins, and is worked when the knee is bent at about 90 degrees.

THE GLUTEAL MUSCLES

There are three separate muscle groups around the backside, collectively known as the gluteals: they are gluteus maximus, gluteus medius and gluteus minimus.

Gluteus maximus is the largest, strongest muscle and is largely responsible for the size and shape of the backside. It attaches to the lower vertebrae and top of the rear part of the pelvis, and inserts into the top third of the back of the femur (thigh bone). Its function is to extend the hip in movements such as squatting, stair climbing and rear leg raises.

Gluteus medius is a smaller muscle, attaching at the top of the rear part of the pelvis and inserting at the top of the femur. Its function is to abduct the hip (move the legs out sideways) and also rotate the hip inwards, so it is used on the leg abductor machine or when doing leg raises to the side.

Gluteus minimus is the smallest of the three gluteals, attaching just below the gluteus medius and inserting at the top of the femur. It tends to act as a stabilising muscle, working eccentrically during impact movements such as running and jumping, and holding the hip joint in position.

THE HIP FLEXORS

The main hip flexors are the iliacus, psoas (ilo-psoas), rectus femoris, pectineus and tensor fascia latae. The iliacus and psoas muscles cannot be seen as they lie deep in the abdomen, running from the lower vertebrae to the top of the thigh bone. They flex the hip. The psoas muscles also help to stabilise the lower back. One of the quadriceps group of muscles, the rectus femoris, runs down the front of the thigh and crosses both the hip joint and the knee joint. It flexes the hip as well as the knee. The pectineus is a short muscle located close to the groin. It is partly covered by the rectus femoris. The tensor fascia latae can be seen on the outer front part of the hip. It helps to flex the hips as well as move the leg outwards.

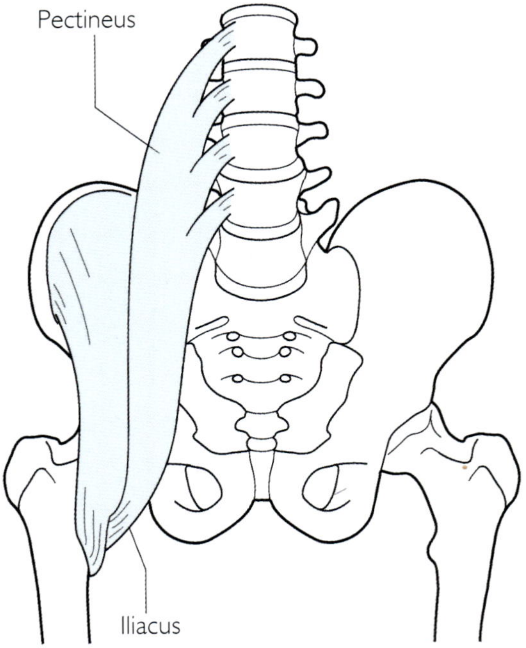

Figure 9.3 The hip flexors

Squat

Target muscles

Gluteals, quadriceps, hamstrings, lower back, adductors, hip flexors

The squat is one of the most efficient exercises for increasing mass, strength and power in the lower body. It is a compound movement that engages many stabiliser muscles in order to complete the lift.

Starting position

1. Position the bar across the upper part of your back so it is resting on your trapezius muscles (not your neck), or hold a pair of dumbbells by your sides (one at each side).
2. Firmly grip the bar, with your hands placed almost double shoulder-width apart. As you lift the bar off the rack, ensure that there is a normal curve (neutral alignment) in your lower back.
3. Position your feet shoulder-width apart (or slightly wider), toes angled out at 30 degrees.

The movement

1. Keeping your head up and your body erect, slowly lower yourself down until your thighs are parallel to the ground; it is not wise to go any further than this. Keep your knees aligned over your feet, pointing in the direction of your toes. Hold this position for a count of 1.
2. From here, press the weight up, pushing hard through your feet and keeping your body erect as you return to the starting position.

Tips

- You should maintain the natural curve in your back throughout the movement.
- If you lack ankle flexibility, it's better to work on this to improve your ROM rather than to use a board under your heels. This is potentially dangerous for the knees because it moves the knees forwards over the feet and can actually reduce your flexibility.
- Breathe in as you lower the weight, allowing your chest to expand and pulling your tummy button in towards your spine. Exhale as you push upwards.

- Keep your eyes fixed on a point in front of you at about eye level.
- Make sure you do not bend forwards excessively or curve your back as this will stress your lower back and reduce the emphasis on your legs.
- Keep your hips under the bar as much as possible and your knees tracking over your toes as you rise.
- Do not rely on a weight belt unless you are using maximal weight or it could result in a weakening of the abdominal muscles. The abdominal wall should be drawn in towards the spine, not pushing against a belt, when lifting.

Variations
Wider stance
Placing your feet just over shoulder-width apart (but not too far or you may lose stability) and taking the squat slightly deeper than parallel places more emphasis on the gluteals on the upward part of the movement. Make sure you practise perfect form and control the squat – you will have to reduce the weight on the bar since going deeper can put greater strain on the knees. You'll find this technique will not only increase your overall strength but will also shape your gluteals!

Smith machine squats
Squats performed using a Smith machine are less effective than barbell squats and may increase injury risk later, when you are not using a machine, as it does not develop the stabiliser muscles. Since the bar travels in a straight line it alters your natural movement, taking much of the emphasis away from your all-important stabilising muscles. If you must use a Smith machine, position your feet so that your heels are directly under the bar.

Front squat

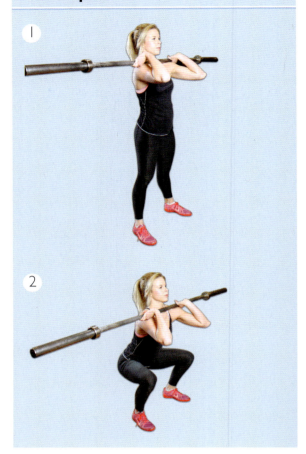

Target muscles
Gluteals, quadriceps, hamstrings, lower back, adductors, hip flexors

The front squat is a variation of the basic, or back, squat where the barbell rests on your front shoulders instead of on your upper back. By pulling the body forward and increasing knee flexion as you descend into a squat, front squats place more of the load on the quadriceps rather than the glutes, hamstrings and lower back.

Starting position
1. Rest the bar across your front deltoids using either an Olympic or cross-arms grip.
2. Position your feet shoulder-width apart (or slightly wider), toes pointing forward.

The movement
1. Squat down, lowering your body until your thighs are just past parallel.
2. Keep your chest lifted, elbows high and knees travelling forward in the same direction as your feet.
3. From here, push through the heel and mid foot and extend the hips and knees simultaneously as you return to the starting position.

Tips
- You should maintain an upright torso and neutral spine throughout the movement.
- Focus on your core to prevent your torso falling forward.
- Since front squats require more skill than back squats to master, use lighter weights than you would for back squats.
- Make sure you keep your heels on the ground.

Split squat

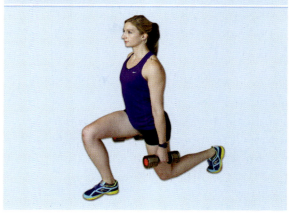

Target muscles
Gluteals, hamstrings, quadriceps

Starting position
1. Position the bar of a Smith machine across the upper part of your back so it is resting on your trapezius muscles (not your neck). Alternatively, hold a pair of dumbbells at your sides (one at each side) with your palms facing your body.
2. Take a step forwards with your right leg and a step back with your left. Your left heel will lift off the floor. The bar should be midway between your two feet.

The movement
1. Drop your body downwards, bending your right knee to 90 degrees, bringing your rear knee to a point just above the floor.

Tips
- When descending, think about dropping your hips straight down so that you avoid bending forwards.

- Keep your head level, your chest out and your back straight.
- Keep your front knee positioned directly over your ankle – do not allow it to extend further forwards.

Variation
On a block
Put your rear foot on a block, step or BOSU which is about 15 cm high. This increases the range of motion and you will feel a greater stretch in the quadriceps of the rear leg.

Dead lift

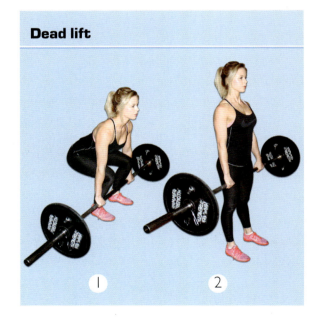

Target muscles
Gluteus maximus, quadriceps, hamstrings, hip flexors, lower back, adductors, latissimus dorsi, trapezius, abdominals

The dead lift is a fundamental exercise for increasing overall mass, strength and power in both the lower and upper body. Like squats, it is a maximum-stimulation movement.

Starting position
1. Stand in front of the barbell with your feet parallel and shoulder-width apart.
2. Bend your legs until your hips and knees are at the same level, keeping your ribcage up and your head level. Your back should be straight, at a 45-degree angle to the floor.
3. Grasp the bar, with your hands just over shoulder-width apart, one overhand, the other under. This will facilitate better balance and keep the barbell in the same plane.

The movement
1. Using the power of your legs and hips, and keeping your arms straight, lift the bar from the floor until your legs are straight. The bar should rest against the upper part of your thighs. Hold for a count of 1.
2. Slowly return the bar to the floor, keeping your torso erect, arms straight and head up, eyes looking forwards. Your chest should be slightly forwards and over the bar.

Tips
- Maintain the normal curvature of your spine throughout the movement – do not lean forwards or tilt backwards.
- Keep your abdominals and lower back muscles contracted to support your spine.
- Drive the movement from your hip muscles – make sure you don't pull with the arms.
- Keep the bar as close as possible to your legs throughout the movement.
- Make sure your knees travel in line with your toes – do not allow them to travel inwards.

Leg press

Target muscles

Gluteals, quadriceps, hamstrings

Also a good strength and mass builder for the lower body, the leg press is often preferred by those with weak lower-back muscles. There is little involvement of the stabiliser muscles and this, paradoxically, may lead to further weakening or imbalance of the deep muscles close to the spine and pelvis. To reduce injury risk, keep your lower back flat on the support.

Starting position

1. Sit into the base of the leg press machine (seated, lying or incline) with your back firmly against the padding.
2. Position your feet parallel and hip-width apart on the platform.
3. Release the safety bars and extend your legs.

The movement

1. Slowly bend your legs and lower the platform in a controlled fashion until your knees almost touch your chest. Hold for a count of 1.
2. Return the platform to the starting position, pushing hard through your heels.

Tips

- Keep your back in full contact with the base; do not allow your lower spine to curl up as you lower the platform.
- Keep your knees in line with your toes.
- Do not 'snap out' or lock your knees as you straighten back to the starting position.
- Make sure you do not bounce your knees off your chest.

Variations

Wide foot spacing

Placing your feet shoulder-width apart, with your toes angled outwards, puts more emphasis on the inner thigh muscles and will therefore help to develop this part of the thigh.

Feet higher on platform

Placing your feet higher on the platform, so that your toes are almost off the edge, puts more emphasis on the hamstrings and gluteals, and will therefore help develop these muscles.

Leg extension

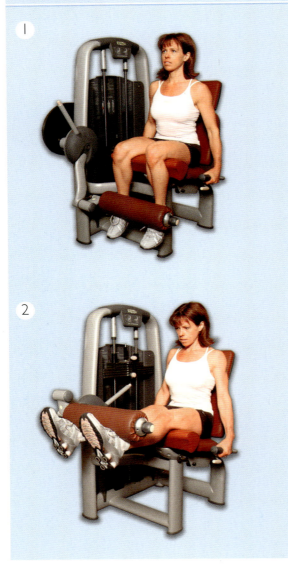

Target muscles
Quadriceps

This exercise helps to develop the front thigh muscles, particularly the 'teardrop' muscles that hold the knee.

Starting position
1. Sit on the leg extension machine, adjusting it so that the backs of your thighs are fully supported on the seat.
2. Hook your feet under the foot pads. The pads should rest on the lowest part of your shins, just above your ankles.
3. Hold on to the sides of the seat or the handles on the sides of the machine to prevent your hips lifting as you perform the exercise.

The movement
1. Straighten your legs to full extension, keeping your thighs and backside fully in contact with the bench.
2. Hold this fully contracted position for a count of 2. Slowly return to the starting point.

Tips
- Do not allow your hips to raise off the seat.
- Try to 'resist' the weight as you lower your legs back to the starting point – avoid letting the weight swing your legs back.
- Make sure you fully straighten the leg until the knees are locked – do not perform partial movements.
- Avoid swinging or kicking your legs – control the movement.

Front lunge

Target muscles
Quadriceps, hamstrings, gluteals

Starting position
1. Hold a pair of dumbbells at the sides of your body with arms fully extended (palms facing your body) or place a bar across the back of your shoulders.
2. Stand with your feet shoulder-width apart, toes pointing forwards. Look straight ahead.

The movement
1. Take an exaggerated step forwards with your right leg, bending the knee, lowering your hips.
2. Lower yourself until your right thigh is parallel to the floor and your knee is at an angle of 90 degrees. Your left leg should be about 10–15 cm above the floor. Hold for a count of 1.
3. Push hard with your right leg to return to the starting position.
4. Complete the desired number of repetitions, then repeat with the left leg leading.

Tips
- Keep your front knee positioned directly over your ankle – do not allow it to extend further forwards as this can cause strain to the knee.
- Keep your body erect throughout the movement – do not lean forwards.

Variation
Step length
A shorter step forwards places more emphasis on the quadriceps; a larger step forwards places more emphasis on the gluteal and hamstring muscles.

Reverse lunge

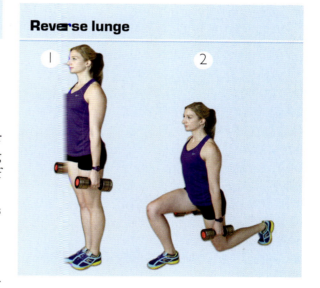

Target muscles
Gluteals, hamstrings, quadriceps

Starting position
1. Place a barbell across the back of your shoulders or hold a pair of dumbbells at the sides of your body
2. Stand with your feet shoulder-width apart, toes pointing forwards.

The movement

1. Drop your right leg behind your body, bending your left leg, lowering your hips and keeping your trunk upright.
2. Lower yourself into a one legged squat position on your left leg until your left thigh is parallel to the floor. Your left knee should be at an angle of 90 degrees. Hold for a count of 1.
3. Push hard through your left leg, strongly contracting the gluteals, quadriceps and hamstrings to return your right leg into position. Make sure you don't push through your right (back) leg.
4. Complete the desired number of repetitions, then repeat with the left leg leading.

Tips

- Keep your front knee positioned directly over your ankle – do not allow it to extend further forwards.
- Keep your body erect and your spine in its neutral position throughout the movement – do not lean forwards and do not round your lower back.
- Make sure you step back far enough so that when you lower your body, the knee of your front leg doesn't pass your toes. In the bottom position, your shin should be vertical.

Walking lunge

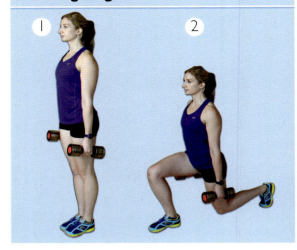

Target muscles
Quadriceps, hamstrings, gluteals

Starting position
1. Hold a pair of dumbbells at the sides of your body, one in each hand, or place a bar across the back of your shoulders.
2. Stand with your feet shoulder-width apart, toes pointing forwards. Look straight ahead.

The movement
1. Take an exaggerated step forwards with your right leg, bending the knee, lowering your hips.
2. Drop your body so your right thigh is parallel to the floor and your left knee is almost touching the floor.
3. Stand back up on your right leg then lunge forward with your left leg.
4. Repeat by alternating lunge with opposite legs.

Tips
- Keep your front knee positioned directly over your ankle – do not allow it to extend further forwards as this can cause strain to the knee.
- Keep your body upright throughout the movement – do not lean forwards.
- The longer your lunge, the more emphasis is placed on the gluteus maximus. A shorter lunge emphasises the quadriceps.

Dumbbell step-ups

Target muscles
Quadriceps, gluteals, hamstrings

Starting position
1. Stand holding a pair of dumbbells, facing a step that is approximately 30–45 cm high.

The movement
1. Step up on to the step with one foot then the other.
2. Step down with the second leg then the first.
3. Repeat with the second leg leading.

Tips
- Do not allow your body to lean forwards while stepping up.
- Make sure your foot is securely on top of the step when you step up.
- Increase the height of the step to work your muscles harder.

Seated leg curl

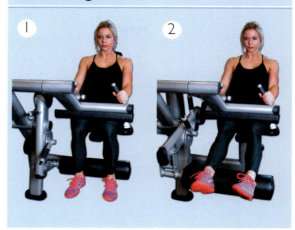

Target muscles
Hamstrings
Also used: gastrocnemius

Starting position
1. Sit down in the leg curl machine and place your heels over the roller pads. Adjust the machine if necessary so that your knees are just off the end of the bench and your thighs fully supported.
2. Hold on to the hand grips or the edge of the bench for support.

The movement
1. Bend your knees, bringing your heels towards your backside.
2. Hold this fully contracted position for a count of 2, then slowly lower your heels back to the starting position.

Tip
- Control the movement on both the upwards and downwards phase; avoid kicking your heels back fast.

Straight leg dead lift

Target muscles
Hamstrings, gluteals, lower back

This exercise requires a high degree of technical skill and flexibility so is unsuitable for beginners and anyone with lower-back problems. When performed correctly, it can work the hamstrings even more effectively than the leg curl.

Starting position
1. Grasp a barbell with your hands slightly wider than shoulder-width apart, using an overhand grip.
2. Stand up straight, looking directly ahead.

The movement
1. Keep your back flat and legs nearly straight.
2. Bend forwards from the hips until your back is parallel to the floor. You should feel a stretch in your hamstrings and gluteals. As you bend forwards, your hips and gluteals should move backwards and your body should be centred through your heels.
3. At the bottom of the movement, do not allow the weight to touch the floor and do not round your back.
4. Hold for a count of one, then forcefully contract your gluteals and hamstrings to raise your torso back to the erect starting position.

Tips
- Keep your back flat. Rounding your back will increase the risk of injury.
- Do not lower the bar too far. The bar should be hanging at arm's length below you, at about knee level. Going below this point hyperflexes the spine, putting it in a vulnerable position and increasing injury risk to the lower back.
- Concentrate on using your hips as a hinge.

Standing calf raise

Target muscles
Gastrocnemius, soleus

This is perhaps the best exercise for overall development of the calves.

Starting position
1. Place your shoulders under the pads of a standing calf raise machine or Smith machine. Alternatively, place a barbell across the back of your shoulders, resting on your trapezius muscles (not your neck).
2. Step on to the platform or, if you are using a barbell, use a step or block. Allow your heels to hang off the edge.
3. Stand with your feet hip-width apart and pointing directly ahead.
4. Straighten your legs as you lift the selected weight clear of the rest of the stack.

The movement
1. Rise up on your toes as high as possible.
2. Hold the fully contracted position for a count of 2, then slowly lower your heels as far as they will go.

Tips
- Keep your legs straight (but not locked) throughout the movement to keep maximal emphasis on the calves and reduce the involvement of the quadriceps.
- Maintain a tight, naturally vertical plane, keeping the natural arch in your back, and your head and neck in a neutral position.
- Stretch your calves fully at the bottom of the movement – your heels should be lower than your toes.
- Do not bounce up from the bottom – keep the movement smooth and continuous.

On toes vs toes in/out
Contrary to popular belief, performing a calf raise with rotated feet (i.e. pointing outwards or inwards) doesn't add any stimulation to particular areas of the calf muscles and may put undue stress on your knee and hip joints. The calf muscles' main function is to plantar flex the foot and this action has little to do with the angle of the feet. Keeping your feet straight therefore maximises calf stimulation and reduces injury risk.

Dumbbell single leg calf raise

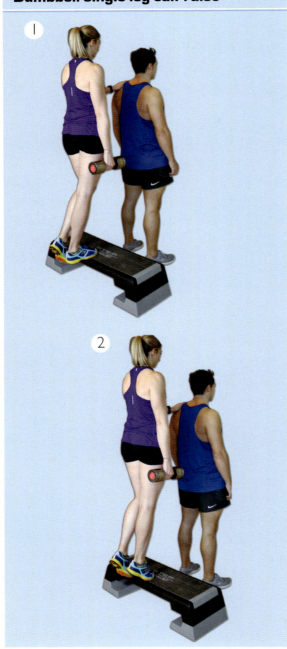

Target muscles
Gastrocnemius, soleus

This exercise is similar to that on a standing calf raise machine but is done one leg at a time.

Starting position
1. Hold a dumbbell in your right hand with your arm hanging down by your side, palm facing your body.
2. Place the ball of the right foot on the edge of a block or platform, allowing your heel to hang off the edge.
3. Hold on to a suitable support with the other hand to steady yourself.

The movement
1. Rise up on the ball of your foot as high as possible.
2. Hold the fully contracted position for a count of 2, then slowly lower your heel as far as it will go.
3. Complete the desired number of repetitions, then repeat on the left leg.

Tips
- Keep your exercising leg straight throughout the movement.
- Keep your body upright.
- Stretch your calf fully at the bottom of the movement – your heel should be lower than your toes.
- Keep the movement smooth and continuous.

Calf (or toe) press

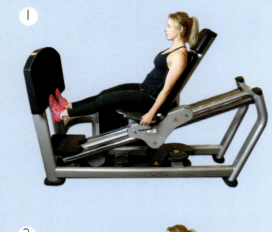

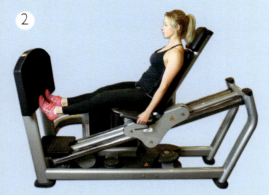

Target muscles
Gastrocnemius, soleus

Starting position
1. Position yourself in a leg press machine.
2. Place the balls of your feet on the bottom of the platform with your heels hanging off the edge. Your legs should be fully extended and feet hip-width apart. Release the safety catch.

The movement
1. Press the platform away from you as far as possible.
2. Hold the fully contracted position for a count of 2, then slowly lower your heels as far as they will go.

Tips
- Stretch your calves fully at the bottom of the movement.
- Keep your legs straight (not locked) throughout the movement.

// THE BACK

10

Training your back will change the proportions of your entire body. Well-developed latissimus dorsi muscles (lats) create that classic V-shape, making your waist appear smaller and, for women, balancing the curves of the lower body.

Strong back muscles are important in sports that involve pulling actions, such as rowing. These actions are used in rugby tackling, judo, boxing, gymnastics and swimming, especially butterfly and front crawl. A strong back will also help you develop other major muscle groups, as your back assists in key exercises such as squatting, shoulder presses and standing biceps curls; while having a strong back helps in everyday activities, such as lifting and carrying, and prevents back injuries.

EXERCISES FOR THE UPPER BACK

Lat pull-down
Pull-up/chin-up
One arm dumbbell row
Seated cable row
Bent-over barbell row
Straight arm pull-down
Machine row
Dumbbell pull-over
Dumbbell shrug

EXERCISES FOR THE LOWER BACK

Back extension (hyperextension) on the floor
Back extension (hyperextension) on the bench
Back extension (hyperextension) on exercise ball
Superman

MUSCLE KNOW-HOW

The major muscles in the upper back include: the trapezius, the diamond-shaped muscle that extends from the back of the neck to the mid back (this may be divided into upper and mid portions) and draws the shoulder blades backwards and upwards, as well as turning the head and bending it backwards; the latissimus dorsi ('lats'), the large wing-like muscles running from your shoulders to your waist that make up the majority of the muscle mass of the upper and mid back, and which draw the arms downwards; the rhomboids (lying beneath the mid part of the trapezius in the central upper back), which help draw the shoulder blades backwards; and the smaller infraspinatus, supraspinatus, teres major and teres minor muscles, which are located around the shoulder blades and rotate the arms outwards.

The erector spinae running along the sides of the mid and lower spine straighten the trunk from a flexed position, as well as moving the trunk sideways. They work in concert with the abdominals and oblique muscles to stabilise the torso.

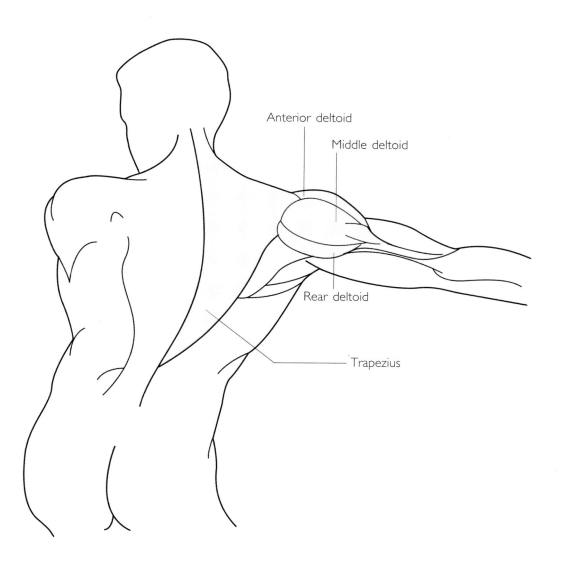

Figure 10.1 Muscles of the back

STRENGTH TRAINING

Lat pull-down

1

2

Target muscles
Latissimus dorsi, rhomboids
  Also used: biceps, posterior deltoids, forearms

Starting position
1. Hold the bar, with your hands just over shoulder-width apart and palms facing forwards.
2. Sit on the seat, adjusting it so that your knees fit snugly under the roller pads. Your arms should be fully extended.

The movement
1. Pull the bar down towards your chest until it touches the upper part of your chest, arching your back slightly.
2. Hold for a count of 2, then slowly return to the starting position.

Tips
- Keep your trunk as still as possible – avoid swinging backwards.
- Focus on keeping your elbows directly under the bar and squeezing your shoulder blades together.
- Do not shorten the return phase of the movement – extend your arms fully.
- Do not lean back too far.

Variations
Close grip
This variation works the inner portion of the latissimus dorsi, thus creating more depth to the mid back. Use a triangle bar attachment and bring it down in front of your neck until it just touches the midpoint of your chest.

Reverse grip
This variation also thickens the latissimus dorsi rather than widening them, thus creating more depth to the mid back. Use a short, straight bar attachment and hold the bar with your palms facing you, about 15–20 cm apart.

Behind neck pull-downs

The front pull-down is considered a better exercise than behind neck pull-downs; researchers at the University of Miami found that it produces a more powerful contraction in the muscles. In addition, pulling the bar down behind the neck increases the potential for injury to the shoulder joint and the upper spine. For this reason, you should pull the bar to your chest, not behind your neck. Still use the other grips from time to time for variety.

Pull-up/chin-up

Target muscles

Latissimus dorsi, trapezius, rhomboids, infraspinatus, teres major and minor

Also used: biceps, posterior deltoids, forearms

Starting position

1. Hold the bar with an overhand (pull-up) or underhand (chin-up) grip, just over shoulder-width apart.
2. Your arms should be fully extended and your ankles crossed to prevent your body from swinging around. If you are using a pull-up machine, place your feet on the platform.

The movement

1. Pull up slowly until your eyes are level with the bar. Lead with your upper chest.
2. Pause for a second or two, then slowly lower back to the starting position.

Tips

- Do not swing your legs forwards or jerk as you pull yourself up – this greatly reduces the stress placed on the back muscles.
- Fix your eyes slightly upwards as you pull yourself up, arching your back just a little.
- Ensure your trunk and thighs maintain a straight line.
- Do not shorten the return phase of the movement – extend your arms fully.

Variation
Close grip

This variation places more stress on the lower lats and biceps. Use either an overhand or underhand grip, with your hands shoulder-width apart.

One arm dumbbell row

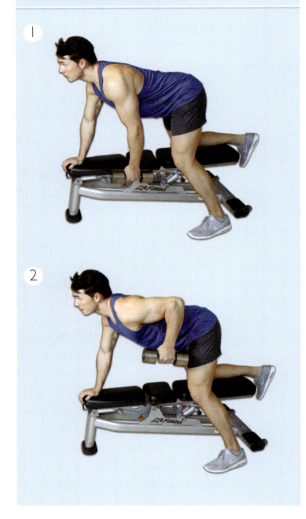

Target muscles
Latissimus dorsi, trapezius, rhomboids, infraspinatus, teres major and minor

Also used: biceps, posterior deltoids

Starting position
1. Hold a dumbbell in your right hand, palm facing your body.
2. Bend forwards from the hips, placing your left hand and knee on a bench to stabilise yourself. Your back should be flat and almost horizontal, and your right arm fully extended.

The movement
1. Pull the dumbbell up towards your waist, drawing your elbow back as far as it can go. Keep the dumbbell close to your body.
2. Allow the dumbbell to touch your ribcage lightly. Pause for a count of 1, then lower the dumbbell slowly until your arm is fully extended.
3. After completing the required number of repetitions, perform the exercise with your left arm.

Tips
- Keep your lower back flat and still – do not twist your trunk.
- Make sure you row the dumbbell to the side of your ribcage – do not pull it up to your shoulder.

Seated cable row

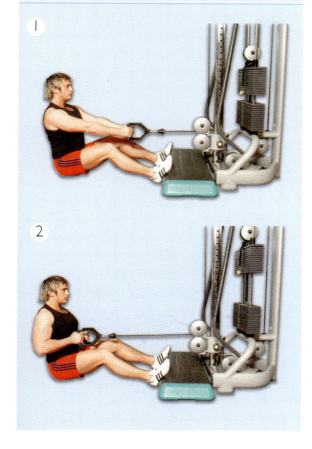

Target muscles
Latissimus dorsi, trapezius, rhomboids, teres major and minor

Also used: erector spinae, biceps, forearms, pectoralis major

Starting position
1. Sit facing the cable row machine and place your feet against the footrests. Grasp the bar and bend your knees slightly.
2. Lean forwards and grasp the pulley handles, while maintaining a normal, slightly curved spinal position.
3. Pull back a little way until your torso is nearly upright and your arms extended fully.

The movement
1. Pull the bar towards you until it touches your lower rib/upper abdomen region. You should be pulling your elbows and shoulders directly backwards as far as possible.
2. Hold for a count of 2, then return slowly to the starting position, maintaining a near-upright position.

Tips
- To achieve maximum back development, keep your torso nearly upright during the entire movement – it should not move forwards or backwards more than 10 degrees.
- Maintain a normal curve in your back – do not arch your back excessively.
- Keep your legs slightly bent and still throughout the movement.
- Inhale at the start of the movement, then hold your breath during the pulling phase – this helps stabilise your torso. Exhale only towards the end of the movement once your arms are extended.

Variation
Straight bar
Cable rows may be performed using a short, straight bar instead of a triangle bar, with a palms-down grip. This emphasises the posterior deltoids, rhomboids and mid part of the trapezius.

Bent-over barbell row

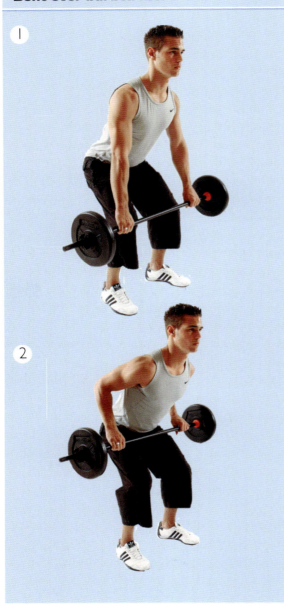

Target muscles
Latissimus dorsi, trapezius, rhomboids, teres major and minor

Also used: biceps, forearms

Starting position
1. Place the bar on the floor in front of you.
2. Stand with your feet parallel and shoulder-width apart.
3. Bending forwards from the hips, keeping your back flat and slightly bending your knees, grasp the bar with an overhand grip slightly wider than shoulder-width apart.
4. Lift the bar just a short way off the floor. Position your body so that your torso is nearly parallel to the ground, arms fully extended.

The movement
1. Slowly pull the bar towards your lower chest until it just touches the lower part of your ribcage.
2. Hold this position for a count of 1, then slowly lower the bar to the starting position.

Tips
- As you pull the bar up, squeeze your shoulder blades together and keep your elbows directly above your hands.
- Keep your back flat throughout the movement – do not round it or you risk injury.
- Keep your torso still – it is tempting to move your torso upwards with the bar to generate momentum. This reduces the work on the back muscles and increases the risk of injury.

Straight arm pull-down

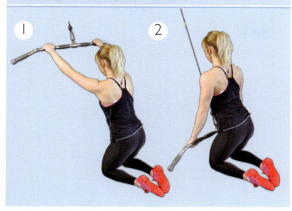

Target muscles
Latissimus dorsi, trapezius, rhomboids, teres major and minor

Starting position
1. Kneel in front of a lat pull-down machine.
2. Hold the bar with your arms extended, palms facing downwards.
3. Pull down the bar to shoulder level.

The movement
1. Keeping your arms extended, pull the bar down until it just touches your upper thighs.
2. Hold for a count of 2, then slowly return the bar to the starting position.

Tips
- Keep your wrists straight throughout the movement.
- Allow a very slight bend in the elbows – they should not be locked.
- Keep your body still and upright throughout the movement – you will need to use your abdominal muscles to stabilise your torso.

Machine row

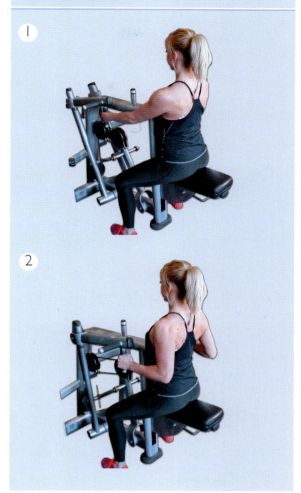

Target muscles
Latissimus dorsi, trapezius, rhomboids, teres major and minor
   Also used: biceps, forearms

Starting position
1. Sit with your chest against the support pad and take an overhand grip on the handles.

The movement
1. Pull the handles towards your sides.
2. Hold for a moment then slowly lower the weight and repeat.

Tips
- Maintain the natural curve in your lower back throughout the movement.
- Don't allow the weight stack to touch down between reps.

Dumbbell pull over

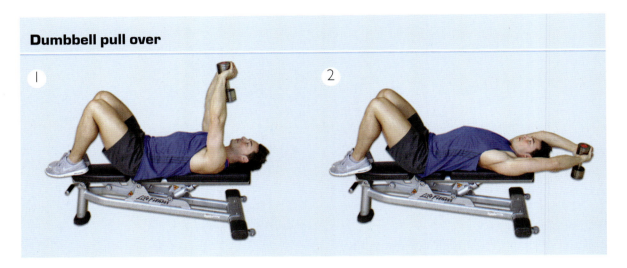

Target muscles
Latissimus dorsi, pectoralis major, triceps

Starting position
1. Lie down perpendicular with just your upper back and shoulders on a flat bench. Your feet should be flat on the floor.
2. Cup your hands around one end of a dumbbell (your palms flat against the top inner plate). Hold the dumbbell over your head with your arms extended.

The movement
1. Slowly lower the dumbbell in a backward arc, down and behind your head, keeping a slight bend in your arms throughout, until your elbows are level with your ears.
2. Raise the dumbbell back over your head using the same arcing motion.

Tips
- Keep your hips lower than your shoulders.
- Avoid arching your back at any time during the movement.
- Don't take the dumbbell back too far – going too deep will increase the risk of incurring a shoulder injury.

Dumbbell shrug

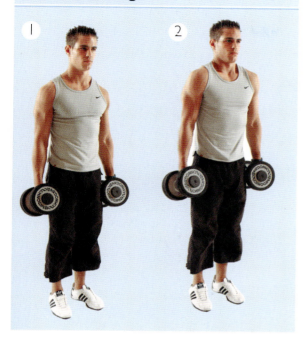

Target muscles
Trapezius (upper), rhomboids, various other neck and shoulder girdle muscles

Starting position
1. Stand with your feet hip-width apart.
2. Hold a pair of dumbbells by your sides level with your thighs, palms facing backwards. Keep your arms straight.

The movement
1. Raise your shoulders straight up towards your ears, keeping your arms straight.
2. Hold for a count of 2, then lower the dumbbells back to the starting position.

Tips
- Keep your arms straight throughout the movement.
- Lift and lower the dumbbells slowly and deliberately – don't jerk them.
- As you lower the dumbbells, allow your shoulders to drop down as far as possible – this stretches the trapezius and increases the ROM.
- Do not rotate your shoulders backwards at the top of the movement – this increases the risk of injury to the shoulder and places no further work on the trapezius.
- Use straps to improve your grip.

Variation
Barbell shrug

Shrugs may be performed with a barbell instead of dumbbells. Hold a barbell in front of or behind your thighs, keep your arms straight and move the bar up and down as described above.

Back extension (hyperextension) on the floor

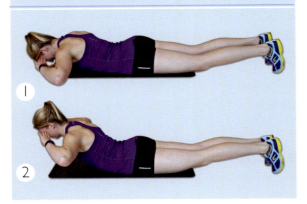

Target muscles
Erector spinae, gluteals

The lower back muscles rarely work through their full ROM during daily activities, nor during exercises for other muscle groups. While the lower back is often involved as a stabiliser in other exercises, such as squats, it is important to include a specific back extension movement in your back workout, which targets the muscles effectively and makes everyday activities easier to perform with less injury risk.

Starting position
1. Lie face down on a mat or the floor.
2. Place your hands by the sides of your head, elbows out to the sides. Alternatively, your arms may be placed behind you, resting on your back.

The movement
1. Slowly raise your head, shoulders and upper chest from the floor. This will be just a short distance.
2. Pause for a count of 2, then lower slowly to the floor.

Tips
- Keep your head facing downwards to the floor in line with your spine.
- Keep your legs relaxed on the floor – do not raise them.
- Only raise yourself as far as is comfortable.

Back extension (hyper extension) on the floor

Target muscles
Erector spinae, gluteals

Starting position
1. Tuck your ankles underneath the pads of a hyperextension bench and position your body so that your hips are resting on the middle pad.
2. Place your hands by the sides of your head or crossed in front of your chest.

The movement
1. Raise your upper body until you are parallel with the floor – do not rise higher than this.
2. Slowly lower your upper body until you are almost perpendicular to the floor.

Tips
- Keep your head facing downwards to the floor in line with your spine.
- Only raise yourself as far as is comfortable.
- To make the movement harder, hold a small weight disc against your chest.

Back extension (hyperextension) on exercise ball

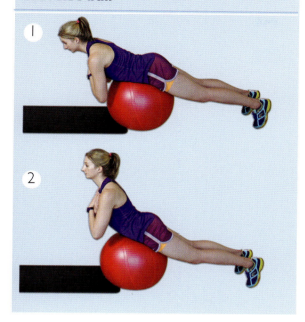

Target muscles
Erector spinae, gluteals

Starting position
1. Lie over an exercise ball, face down, keeping your hips halfway up the ball rather than balanced on top of it. Place your feet against a wall for support if you like.
2. Place your arms either crossed over your chest or by the sides of your head.
3. Keep your legs wide and straight behind you.

The movement
1. Raise your upper body slowly in a straight line towards the ceiling.
2. Hold for a count of 2, then lower again slowly.

Tips
- Do not arch your back.
- Keep your head in line with your spine.
- To make the movement harder, bring your legs closer together.

Superman

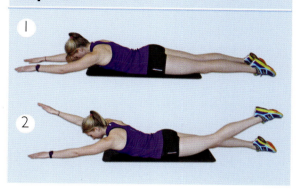

Target muscles
Erector spinae, gluteals

Starting position
1. Lie face down on a mat with your arms stretched out in front of you and your legs straight.

The movement
1. Slowly raise your left arm and your right leg, keeping them both straight. This will be just a short distance.
2. Hold for a count of 2, then lower slowly to the floor. Repeat, raising the opposite arm and leg.

Tips
- Keep your head facing downwards to the floor in line with your spine.
- Only raise as far as you feel comfortable.

THE CHEST

The desire for a bigger, better-developed chest is perhaps the greatest motivator for men to strength train. It somehow symbolises heroism and male virility. Women, too, can benefit from chest training. Although it won't increase the size of your breasts (they are mostly fat tissue), it will create the appearance of a fuller and more shapely chest.

Strong chest muscles are advantageous in many sports. These muscles are involved in all forward- and upward-reaching actions – e.g. in rugby tackling and grabbing an opponent – and are also used in throwing and hitting movements – e.g. during forehand drives in tennis and squash; when throwing the ball overhead in netball, basketball and volleyball; throwing the discus and javelin, and putting the shot. A strong chest is also advantageous in swimming (breaststroke) and several gymnastic disciplines.

EXERCISES FOR THE CHEST

Barbell bench press
Vertical bench press machine
Dumbbell press
Incline barbell bench press
Incline dumbbell bench press
Dumbbell flye
Pec-deck flye
Cable cross-over
Low-pulley cable cross-over

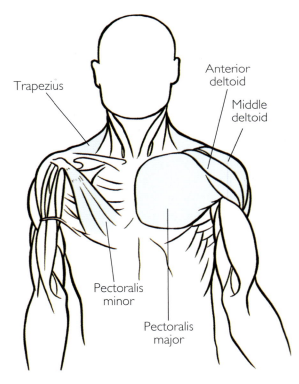

Figure 11.1 Muscles of the chest

MUSCLE KNOW-HOW

The largest muscle of the chest is the pectoralis major, which attaches to the collarbone (clavicle) and sternum, and inserts into the upper arm bone (humerus). It pulls the arm in front of the chest from any position, flexes the shoulder to allow pushing, and lifts the arm forwards. The smaller pectoralis minor lies beneath the pectoralis major and helps lower the shoulder blade.

Barbell bench press

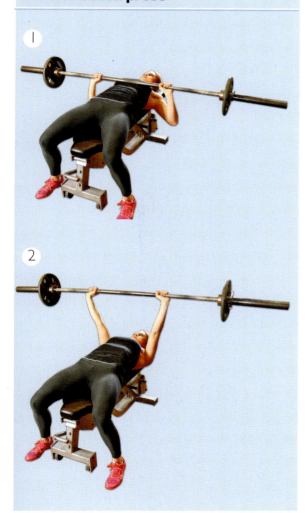

Target muscles
Pectoralis major (mid chest)
   Also used: anterior deltoids, triceps

Starting position
1. Lie on your back on a flat bench, ideally with an attached barbell rack. If you have an excessive arch in your back, place your feet on the end of the bench or on a low step.
2. Hold the bar, with your hands just over shoulder-width apart, palms facing forwards.
3. Remove the bar from the barbell rack and position it directly over your chest with your arms fully extended (but not locked).

The movement
1. Slowly lower the bar down to your chest. The bar should touch your upper chest just above your nipple line. Hold in this position for a count of 2.
2. Push the bar upwards in a slightly backwards arc so that it ends up over your shoulders.

Tips
- Keep your hips firmly on the bench. If you lift your hips to generate leverage, you will risk lower-back strain.
- Do not bounce the bar off your chest or arch your back – this reduces the amount of chest work and risks injury to the chest muscles.
- Keep your palms facing forwards and your wrists straight.

Variations
Wide grip
Using a grip one and a half times shoulder-width apart places more emphasis on the pectorals (especially the outer part) and less on the triceps.

Narrow grip
Using a shoulder-width grip places more emphasis on the triceps and the inner pectorals.

Vertical bench press machine

Target muscles
Pectoralis major
Also used: anterior deltoids, triceps

Starting position
1. Sit down with your back pressed against the backrest.
2. Adjust the seat height so that the handles are level with your chest. Depress the foot lever to allow you to grab hold of the handles.

The movement
1. Press the handles away from you, fully extending your arms.
2. Hold for a second then return slowly to the starting position.

Tip
• Keep your elbows at the same height throughout the movement.

Dumbbell press

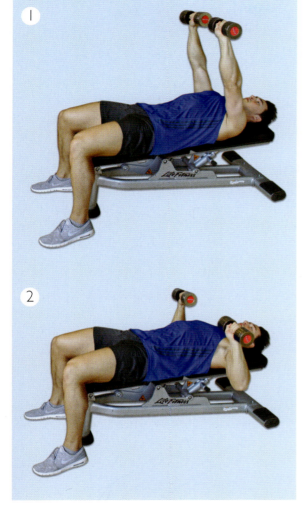

Target muscles
Pectoralis major (mid chest)
  Also used: anterior deltoids, triceps

This exercise develops the chest muscles, but allows a slightly greater ROM compared with the bench press, thus stimulating greater development. It requires more involvement of the stabiliser muscles to balance and control the dumbbells, so you will probably need to use less weight.

Starting position
1. Lie on your back on a flat or incline bench. If you have an excessive arch in your back, place your feet on the end of the bench.
2. Hold a pair of dumbbells, with your palms facing forwards and your arms fully extended, positioned over your shoulders.

The movement
1. Slowly lower the dumbbells down to your armpit area.
2. Hold the position for a count of 2, then press the dumbbells back in to the starting position.

Tips
- Keep your hips firmly on the bench throughout the movement.
- Lower the dumbbells as far as you can, aiming for a maximum stretch but which still feels comfortable.
- Keep the dumbbells over your chest – do not let them travel back towards your head.

Incline barbell bench press

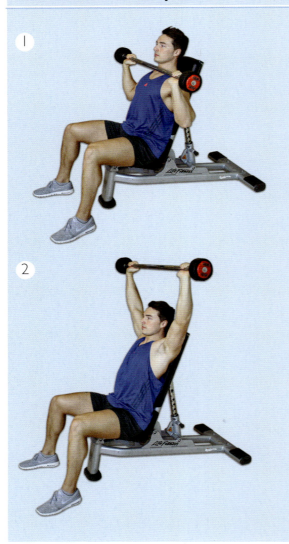

Starting position
1. Lie on an incline bench angled at 30–60 degrees (the steeper the incline, the greater the stress on the upper pectorals and anterior deltoids). Ideally the bench should have an attached barbell rack.
2. Hold the bar with your hands shoulder-width apart, palms facing forwards. Remove the bar from the barbell rack so it is positioned directly over your collarbone with your arms fully extended.

The movement
1. Bend your arms, allowing your elbows to travel out to the sides, and slowly lower the bar down to your chest.
2. The bar should just touch the upper part of your chest beneath your collarbone. Hold for a count of 2.
3. Push the bar back to the starting position.

Tips
- Do not arch your back or bounce the bar off your chest as you push the bar upwards. This risks lower-back strain.
- The higher you place the bar on your chest, the greater the work placed on the anterior deltoids rather than the upper chest.

Variation
Decline
Set the decline bench about 30 degrees below parallel. The movement is the same but places more emphasis on your lower chest and triceps.

Target muscles
Pectoralis minor (upper chest)

Also used: anterior deltoids, triceps, pectoralis major

Incline dumbbell bench press

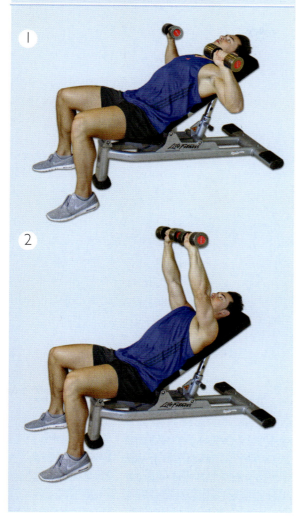

Target muscles
Pectoralis minor (upper chest)

Also used: anterior deltoids, triceps, pectoralis major

Starting position
1. Sit on an incline bench, angled at 30–60 degrees (the steeper the incline, the greater the stress on the upper pectorals and anterior deltoids).
2. Pick up a dumbbell in each hand and place them on your thighs.
3. Lie on the bench, at the same time bringing the dumbbells to shoulder level. Your palms should face forwards.

The movement
1. Press the dumbbells directly over your upper chest until your arms are fully extended. Hold for a count of 2.
2. Lower the weights slowly until they are by your shoulders. You should achieve a maximal but comfortable stretch.
3. Pause for a second before pressing them up over your chest again.

Tips
- Press the dumbbells in a straight line, not back over your head.
- Do not set the angle of the bench too high otherwise the anterior deltoids will be targeted and take much of the emphasis away from the chest.

Dumbbell flye

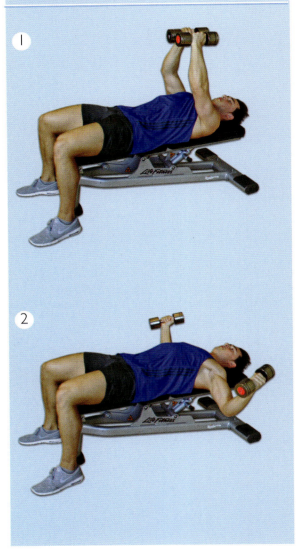

Target muscles
Pectoralis major (mid chest)
Also used: anterior deltoids, pectoralis minor

Starting position
1. Lie on your back on a flat or incline bench set at 30 degrees with your feet flat on the floor. If you have an excessive arch in your back, place your feet on a step so that your knees are bent at 90 degrees.
2. Take a dumbbell in each hand and hold them above your chest with your arms extended and palms facing each other. Bend your arms very slightly.

The movement
1. Lower the dumbbells slowly out to your sides in a semicircular arc. Keep your elbows locked in the slightly bent position throughout the movement.
2. When your upper arms reach shoulder level and you feel a strong stretch in your shoulders, return the dumbbells to the starting position, following the same arc. Do not pause at the bottom of the movement.

Tips
- Maintain the slight bend in your elbows. Don't allow them to bend to 90 degrees as this would turn the movement into a dumbbell press.
- Do not allow your upper arms to go much below shoulder level as this could place excessive stress on the shoulder joints and risk muscle or tendon tears.

Pec-deck flye

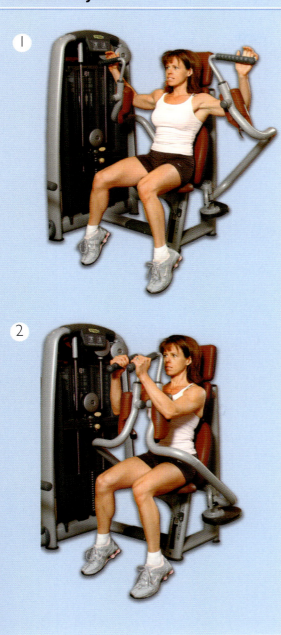

Target muscles
Pectoralis major (mid chest)
   Also used: anterior deltoids, pectoralis minor

Starting position
1. Sit on the seat of the pec-deck machine, ensuring your lower back is pressed against the back support, and adjust the seat height so that your elbows and shoulders are level with the bottom of the pads.
2. Place your forearms against the pads. Check that your shoulders and elbows form a horizontal line.

The movement
1. Move the pads towards each other until they just touch in front of your chest.
2. Hold for a count of 2, then slowly return the pads to the starting position.

Tips
- Contract your pectorals hard when at the midpoint.
- Do not curl your shoulders forwards as you bring the pads together.
- Move the pads in a smooth arc – do not jerk them together as this reduces the work on the pectorals.

Cable cross-over

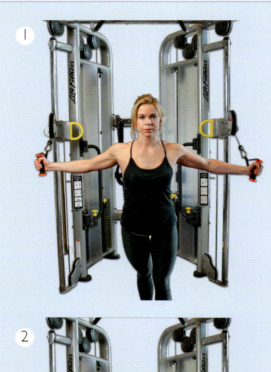

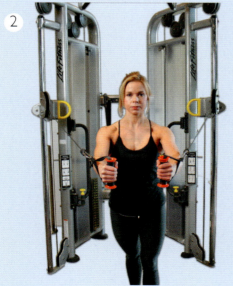

Target muscles
Pectoralis major (lower and mid chest)
Also used: anterior deltoids

Starting position
1. Attach the handles to two overhead pulley machines.
2. Hold the handles, palms facing down, and stand midway between the machines with your feet hip-width apart or with one foot in front of the other for balance. Your arms should be fully extended so you achieve a good stretch in your pectorals.
3. Bend forwards slightly from the hips and keep this position throughout the exercise.

The movement
1. Draw the handles towards each other in an arcing motion, aiming for a point approximately 30 cm in front of your hips.
2. When the handles meet, squeeze your pectorals hard and hold for a count of 2.
3. Return the handles slowly to reach the starting position.

Tips
- Keep your back erect and elbows slightly bent (at 10–15 degrees) throughout.
- Focus on using your chest muscles to perform the movement – do not curl your shoulders forwards as you bring the handles together.
- You can vary the angle at which you pull the handles down to place emphasis on slightly different areas of the chest.

Low-pulley cross-over

Target muscles
Pectoralis major (upper and mid chest), pectoralis minor

Also used: anterior deltoids

Starting position
1. Stand midway between two low-cable machines.
2. Hold the handles with a palms-up grip and stand with your feet hip-width apart or with one foot in front of the other for balance. Your arms should be fully extended so you achieve a good stretch in your pectorals.
3. Bend forwards from the hips at about 10–20 degrees.

The movement
1. Pull your arms in and slightly upwards, bringing your hands up under your chest while keeping your elbows in their slightly bent position.
2. Aim for your hands to meet in front of your abs. Hold for a moment.
3. Slowly return the handles to reach the starting position.

Tips
- Keep your body stationary at all times; the angle in your shoulder should be constant.
- Keep your arms straight, with your elbows slightly bent throughout the movement.

THE CHEST

// THE SHOULDERS

12

Shoulder training can change the proportions of your physique. Well-developed shoulders draw more attention to your upper body and create an aesthetically pleasing taper, making your waist appear smaller.

Strong shoulders are advantageous in most sports involving upper body motions. The shoulder muscles are involved in:

- overhead pushing actions – e.g. tumbling and vaulting in gymnastics, and the clean and jerk in weightlifting
- overhead hitting actions – e.g. the tennis serve, the overhead smash in badminton, and overhead hits and blocks in volleyball and basketball
- raising the arms forwards or sideways away from the body – e.g. tennis or squash strokes, and front crawl in swimming.

You need to use a variety of exercises to train your shoulders as there is no single exercise that works the whole area. The shoulders comprise three heads (see Figure 12.1), each of which needs to be targeted if you want full and well-balanced development.

If you are prone to shoulder injuries, however, pay attention to your training method as

poor technique can exacerbate any underlying problems.

EXERCISES FOR THE SHOULDERS

Shoulder press (dumbbell)
Shoulder press (barbell)
Overhead press machine
Lateral raise
Front lateral raise
Upright row
Bent-over lateral raise

MUSCLE KNOW-HOW

The shoulder muscle comprises three distinct portions, or heads, collectively known as the deltoids. This is a term derived from the Greek 'delta' and reflects their geometrically triangular shape. The deltoids cover the front, side and back of the shoulder, from the scapula (collarbone) to the middle of the upper arm (humerus). Each head serves a particular function. The anterior (front) deltoid lifts the arm forwards and upwards; the medial (outer) deltoid lifts the arm away from the midline of the body to the side (abduction);

and the posterior (rear) deltoid lifts the arm to the rear or draws the elbow backwards behind the shoulders. Because of their location and function, several of the following exercises that target the deltoids also use muscles in the back and chest (see pp. 148 and 150).

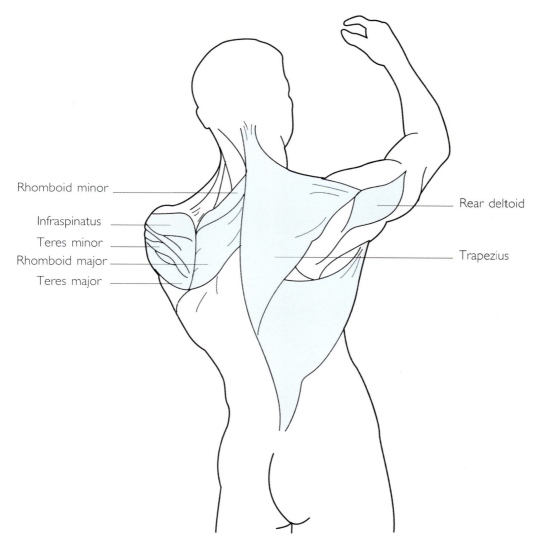

Figure 12.1 Muscles of the shoulders

Shoulder press (dumbbell)

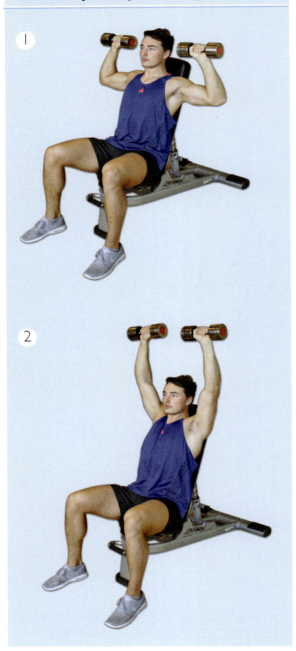

Target muscles
Anterior and medial deltoids, upper pectoralis major

Also used: triceps, shoulder girdle muscles (trapezius, supraspinatus)

Starting position
1. Sit on the edge of a bench or on an exercise ball, angled at 75–90 degrees so that your lower back is firmly in contact with the bench. If you are using a very heavy weight, use an adjustable bench which has an upright back support.
2. Hold a pair of dumbbells, palms facing forwards, level with your shoulders.

The movement
1. Press the dumbbells upwards and inwards until they almost touch over your head.
2. Straighten your arms but do not lock out your elbows. Hold momentarily.
3. Lower the dumbbells slowly back to the starting position.

Tips
- Keep your torso upright – don't lean backwards or arch your spine as you press the bar upwards as this will strain the lower back.
- Hold your abdominal muscles taut to help stabilise your spine.
- Lower the dumbbells until they touch your shoulders – don't shorten the movement.

Shoulder press (barbell)

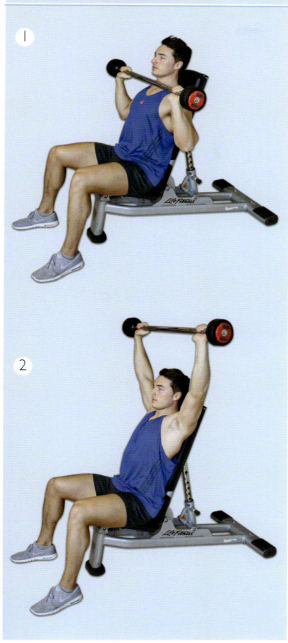

Target muscles
Anterior and medial deltoids, upper pectoralis major

Also used: triceps, shoulder girdle muscles (trapezius, supraspinatus)

Starting position
1. Sit on the edge of a bench, angled at 75–90 degrees so that your lower back is firmly in contact with the bench. If you are using a very heavy weight, use an adjustable bench which has an upright back support.
2. Grasp a barbell with your hands slightly wider than shoulder-width, palms forwards. Position the bar near your upper chest.

The movement
1. Press the barbell upwards until your arms are extended, but not locked out.
2. Hold momentarily, then lower slowly back to the starting position.

Tips
- Keep your torso upright – don't lean backwards or arch your spine as you press the bar upwards as this will strain the lower back.
- Hold your abdominal muscles taut to help stabilise your spine.
- Don't use too wide a grip, otherwise your ROM will be shortened.

Overhead press machine

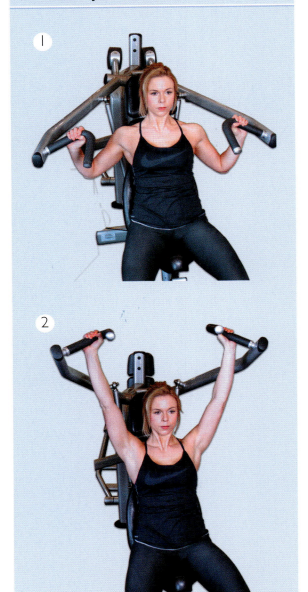

Target muscles
Anterior and medial deltoids, upper pectoralis major

Also used: triceps, shoulder girdle muscles (trapezius, supraspinatus)

Starting position
1. Sit in the machine with your feet on the floor and your back against the backrest. Adjust the seat height so that the handles are level with your shoulders.
2. Depress the foot lever to allow you to grasp the handles more comfortably.

The movement
1. Grip the handles and press the weight straight up, extending your arms but not locking out your elbows.
2. Lower the weight slowly and repeat.

Tip
- Keep your back flat against the pad.

Lateral raise

|

2

Target muscles
Medial deltoids
Also used: trapezius, anterior deltoids

Starting position
1. Stand with your feet hip-width apart. Hold a dumbbell in each hand, arms straight down by your sides, hands facing inwards.

The movement
1. Keeping your elbows very slightly bent (at about 10 degrees), raise the dumbbells out to the sides.
2. Raise them until your elbows and hands are level with your shoulders – i.e. parallel to the floor. Your palms should face the floor. Hold momentarily.
3. Return slowly to the starting position, resisting the weight on the way back down.

Tips
• Your little finger should be higher than your thumb at the top of the movement, as if you were pouring water from a jug.
• Do not swing the dumbbells out or lean back as you raise them. Keep your body very still.
• Lead with your elbows, not your hands.

Variations
Single arm lateral raise
Lateral raises can be performed using one arm at a time. Hold on to an upright support with the other hand to help keep you steady. This allows you to concentrate fully on the movement and helps to prevent you swinging the dumbbells upwards.

Cable lateral raise
The movement can be performed using a low pulley machine. You will need to use a lighter weight but this keeps more continuous tension on the deltoids.

THE SHOULDERS

Front lateral raise

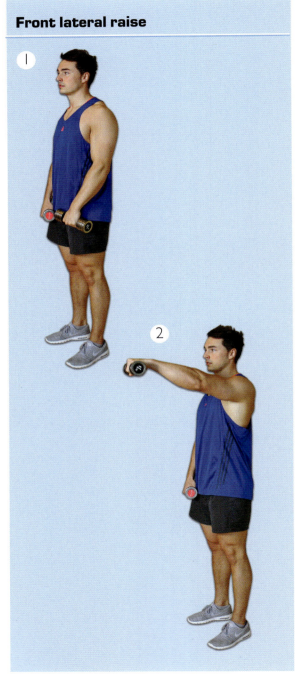

Target muscles
Anterior deltoids

Also used: Medial deltoids, pectoralis major, trapezius

Starting position
1. Stand with your feet hip-width apart. Hold a dumbbell in each hand, positioned in front of your legs with arms straight.

The movement
1. Raise the dumbbells forward and upward until your upper arms are just above horizontal. Your palms should face the floor. Hold momentarily.
2. Return slowly to the starting position.

Tips
- Do not swing the dumbbells. Keep the movement controlled.
- Keep your elbows very slightly bent (at about 10 degrees).
- You may prefer to perform the movement alternating right and left arms.

Upright row

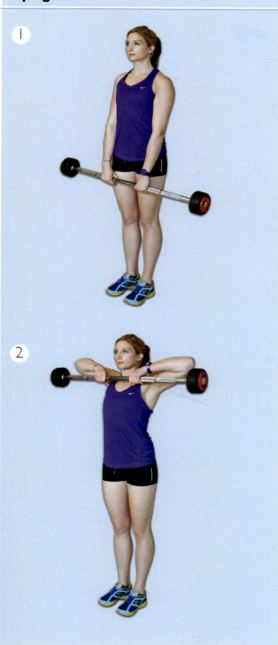

Target muscles
Anterior and medial deltoids, trapezius
Also used: biceps, brachioradialis

Starting position
1. Stand with your feet shoulder-width apart.
2. Hold the barbell with your hands about 15 cm apart, palms facing towards your body. The bar should rest against the front of your thighs. The exercise can also be performed on a cable machine, using a short, straight bar attached to the low pulley.

The movement
1. Pull the bar directly upwards towards your chin, bending your elbows out to the sides until the bar is level with your neck.
2. Hold for a count of 2, then lower the bar slowly back to the starting position.

Tips
- Keep the bar very close to your body throughout the movement.
- Make sure you do not sway backwards as you lift the bar.
- At the top of the movement your elbows should be level with, or slightly higher than, your hands.
- Lower the bar slowly, resisting the weight.

Variation
Wide grip
Using a shoulder-width grip places more emphasis on the deltoids, less on the trapezius.

Bent-over lateral raise

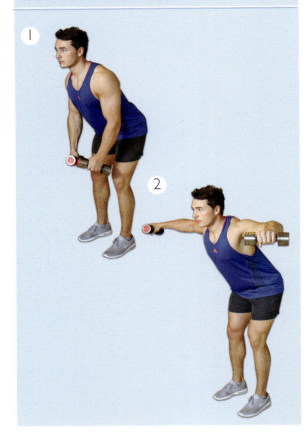

Target muscles
Posterior deltoids
  Also used: trapezius, upper back muscles

Starting position
1. Sit on the end of a bench with only half of your thighs supported.
2. Place your feet and knees together, bend forwards from the waist and hold a pair of dumbbells underneath your thighs with your palms facing each other.

The movement
1. Draw the dumbbells out to the sides, simultaneously turning your hands so that they face the floor.
2. Raise the dumbbells until your elbows and hands are level with your shoulders. Hold momentarily.
3. Slowly return to the starting position, resisting the weight on the way down.

Tips
- Your little finger should be higher than your thumb at the top of the movement, as if you are pouring water from a jug.
- Keep your torso still – do not raise your body as you raise the dumbbells.
- Lead with your elbows, not your hands.
- Keep your elbows bent at about 10 degrees throughout to avoid straining them.

Variation
Standing bent-over lateral raise
The movement can be executed from a standing position. Stand with your feet hip-width apart, bend forwards from the hips and hold the dumbbells directly below the shoulders (arms straight).

Dumbbell lateral raise on incline bench
The movement can be performed face down on an incline bench set at a 30–45 degree angle.

THE ARMS

13

Arms are the classic showpieces of strength for gym-goers. Like a well-developed chest, they are visible proof of the work you put in at the gym. For both men and women, toned, defined arms are enviable assets.

Developing your arm strength will help your performance in many sports. Elbow flexion (bending) and the muscles involved are important when playing forehand strokes in tennis and squash, shooting in hockey, playing a long shot in golf, pulling the body upwards in climbing, grabbing an opponent in rugby and the martial arts, and pushing movements in gymnastics.

The triceps are also involved in numerous upper-body actions, including:

- overhead hitting and throwing movements – e.g. the tennis serve, volleyball spike and basketball shot
- pushing actions – e.g. the shot put, the chest pass in netball and basketball, throwing a punch in boxing and in the martial arts.

One common mistake is to train only the biceps, thinking this will produce stronger and bigger arms. However, the triceps make up the largest part of the arm muscles (see p. 152) so it is important to devote equal time and effort to triceps training. Some also use weights that are too heavy in their quest for bigger arms, sacrificing good technique and therefore gaining only minimal results.

EXERCISES FOR THE ARMS

Barbell curl
Preacher curl
Dumbbell curl
Incline dumbbell curl
Concentration curl
Triceps push-down
Reverse-grip triceps press-down
Bench dip
Lying triceps extension
Triceps kickback
Seated overhead triceps extension

MUSCLE KNOW-HOW

Approximately 60 per cent of the upper-arm muscle mass is comprised of the triceps, 30 per cent is comprised of the biceps brachii, and the remaining 10 per cent comes from the brachialis muscles lying beneath the biceps.

The biceps brachii (see Figure 13.1) originates above the shoulder as two muscles – the short and long heads ('bi' means 'two') – that merge at one insertion point below the elbow. These muscles are involved in flexing your arm (bending your elbow) and rotating (supinating) your forearm. The biceps brachii also assists in other arm and shoulder movements, such as raising the shoulder. The brachialis runs under the biceps close to your elbow joint. It is also involved in arm flexion and all movements involving a palms-down position (e.g. when performing a reverse curl). The brachioradialis lies on the top side of your forearm, on the same side as your thumb but is attached just past your elbow. It is involved in all arm flexion movements, particularly when you use a neutral, or thumbs-up, grip.

The triceps brachii (see Figure 13.2) makes up the entire back of the arm. It has three distinct heads: the inner (long) head, the medial head and outer (lateral) head. The medial head is located on the back inner side of the arm, close to the elbow. The lateral head, which works progressively harder as the weight increases, is located on the back outer side of the arm. The long inner head, lying between the medial and lateral heads higher up on the arm, gives the familiar horseshoe appearance to the outside upper arm. Whereas the medial and lateral heads only cross the elbow joint, the long head crosses both the shoulder and elbow joints.

The collective function of the triceps brachii is, partially or fully, to straighten the arm from a bent position. While it is difficult to isolate its individual heads, different exercises place greater emphasis on different areas. For example, the long head is best stimulated when your arm is raised overhead (e.g. in lying triceps extensions).

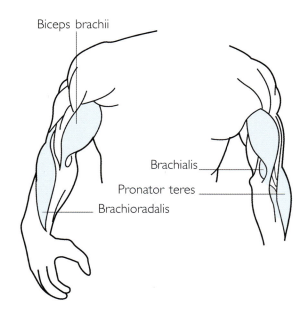

Figure 13.1 Muscles of the front upper arm

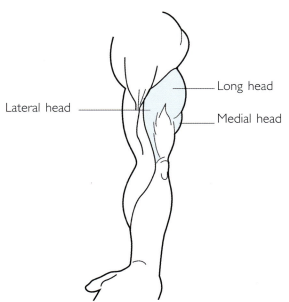

Figure 13.2 Muscles of the back upper arm

Barbell curl

Target muscles

Biceps brachii, brachialis
Also used: brachioradialis

Starting position

1. Stand with your feet hip-width apart.
2. Hold a barbell with your hands shoulder-width apart, palms facing forwards.
3. The bar should rest against your thighs and your arms should be fully extended.

The movement

1. Bend your elbows as you curl the bar up in a smooth arc towards your shoulders. Keep your upper arms fixed by your sides.
2. Hold for a count of 2, then slowly lower the bar back to the starting position.

Tips

- Do not move your upper arms or elbows at any point of the movement.
- Keep your body absolutely still – make sure you do not lean back or swing the bar up as this will strain the back and reduce the work on the biceps.
- Keep your wrists locked.
- Lower the bar under control until your arms are fully extended – shortening or rushing the downward phase will reduce the effectiveness of the exercise.

Variation

EZ-bar curl

Arm curls can be performed using an EZ-bar instead of a straight bar. This reduces the stress on the wrists, although it puts the biceps in a biomechanically weaker position so they receive less stimulation.

STRENGTH TRAINING

Preacher curl

Target muscles
Biceps brachii, brachialis
Also used: brachioradialis

Starting position
1. Adjust the seat on the preacher curl bench to the right height – your armpits should rest over the top edge of the pad. If a preacher bench isn't available, simply use an incline bench and perform the exercise with a dumbbell one arm at a time.
2. Hold a dumbbell or barbell with your hands shoulder-width apart, palms facing forwards.
3. Your arms should be fully extended.

The movement
1. Bend your elbows as you curl the barbell or dumbbell up in a smooth arc towards your shoulders, stopping about 20–30 cm short of your shoulders.
2. Hold for a count of 2, then slowly lower the bar back to the starting position.

Tips
- Keep your shoulders back and relaxed – avoid leaning forwards as you curl the bar up or the emphasis will shift from your biceps to your shoulders.
- Keep your body still and your wrists locked.
- Lower the bar until your arms are fully extended – shortening the downward phase will reduce the effectiveness of the exercise.

Variations
EZ-bar preacher curl
Preacher curls can be performed using an EZ-bar instead of a straight bar. This reduces the stress on the wrists, although it puts the biceps in a biomechanically weaker position so they receive less stimulation.

Dumbbell curl

Target muscles
Biceps brachii, brachialis
Also used: brachioradialis

Starting position
1. Stand with your feet hip-width apart or sit on the end of a bench or on an exercise ball.
2. Hold a pair of dumbbells, palms facing outwards.
3. Your arms should be fully extended.

The movement
1. Curl one dumbbell up at a time in a smooth arc towards your shoulders, rotating your shoulder at the top of the movement.
2. Hold for a count of 2, then slowly lower the dumbbell back to the starting position.
3. Repeat with the other arm and continue alternating arms.

Tips
- Curl the dumbbells up slowly – do not swing them.
- Keep your upper arms fixed by the sides of your body.
- Keep your body absolutely still – make sure you do not sway backwards.
- Make sure you straighten your arms fully when you lower the dumbbells; do not shorten the downward phase.

THE ARMS

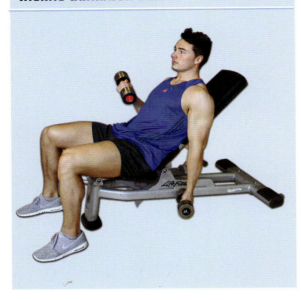

Incline dumbbell curl

The movement
1. Slowly curl one dumbbell towards your shoulder, rotating your forearm so that your palm faces your shoulder at the top of the movement.
2. Hold for a count of 2, then slowly lower the dumbbell back to the starting position.
3. Repeat with the other arm and continue alternating arms.

Tips
- The lower the incline, the greater the stretch on the upper biceps.
- Keep your back against the bench throughout the movement.
- Keep your elbows pointed down and back as best as possible.

Target muscles
Biceps brachii, brachialis
  Also used: brachioradialis

Starting position
1. Sit on an incline bench with your back and shoulders pressed firmly against it.
2. Hold a pair of dumbbells by your sides, palms facing inwards.
3. Your arms should be fully extended and hang downwards.

Concentration curl

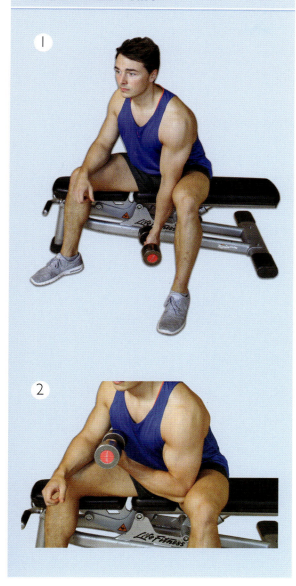

Target muscles
Biceps brachii, brachialis
Also used: brachioradialis

Starting position
1. Sit on a bench with your legs fairly wide apart.
2. Hold a dumbbell with one hand and brace that arm against the inside of the same thigh.
3. Your arm should be fully extended and your palm should be facing the opposite thigh.

The movement
1. Curl the dumbbell up slowly in a smooth arc towards your shoulder.
2. Squeeze your biceps hard at the top of the movement, hold for a count of 2, then slowly lower the dumbbell back to the starting position.

Tips
- Make sure you curl the dumbbell to your shoulder and do not move your shoulder to the dumbbell.
- Keep your shoulder back and relaxed.
- Do not lean backwards.
- Keep your upper arm fixed.
- Make sure you straighten your arms fully when you lower the dumbbells; do not shorten the downward phase.

Triceps push-down

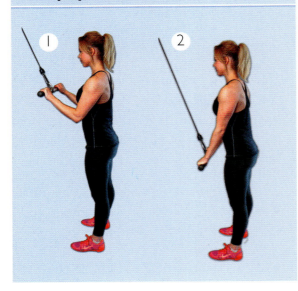

Target muscles
Triceps (especially the outer and medial heads)
Also used: brachioradialis

Starting position
1. Attach a short, angled or straight bar to the overhead cable of a lat machine. Alternatively, use a short rope attachment.
2. Place your hands on the bar, palms facing downwards.
3. Bring the bar down until your elbows are at your sides and bent at about 90 degrees.

The movement
1. Keeping your upper arms close to your body, press the bar down, moving only your forearms, until your arms are fully extended.
2. Hold for a count of 2, then slowly return the bar to the starting position.

Tips
- Keep your elbows fixed firmly at your sides throughout the movement.
- Do not lean too far forwards.
- Keep your wrists locked and your palms facing you.

Reverse-grip triceps press-down

Target muscles
Triceps (especially the lateral head)
Also used: brachioradialis

Starting position
1. Stand in front of a high-pulley cable machine. Position one leg slightly in front of the other.
2. Grasp the stirrup handle palm-up.
3. Bring the bar down until your elbow is bent at an angle of about 90 degrees.

The movement
1. Press the handle down, until your arm is fully extended. Keep your elbow at your side.
2. Hold for a count of 2, then slowly return the handle to the starting position. Repeat for reps then switch arms.

Tips
- Keep your upper arm and elbow locked in to the side of your body.
- Make sure you fully extend your arm and lock out your elbow at the bottom of the press-down.

Variation
This exercise can be performed with a short, straight bar.

Bench dip

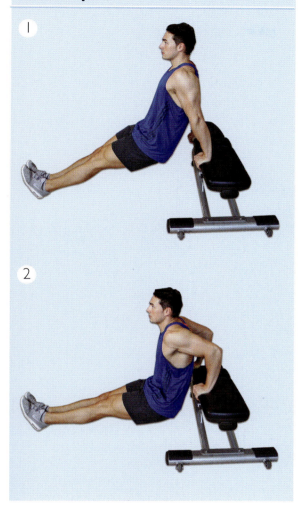

Target muscles
Triceps (especially the outer and medial heads)

Starting position
1. Position two benches or steps about the length of your legs apart.
2. Place your hands shoulder-width apart, fingers facing forwards, on the edge of one bench.
3. Place your heels on the other bench so that your legs form a straight bridge between the two benches.

The movement
1. Bend your elbows and lower your body until your elbows form an angle of 90 degrees.
2. Hold for a count of 2, then straighten your arms to return to the starting position.

Tips
- Keep your back close to the bench.
- Do not lock or snap out your elbows at the top of the movement.
- Keep your elbows directed backwards during both the lowering and raising phases.
- Do not shorten the downward phase.
- Keep the movement slow; do not rush the reps.

Variations
Easier
Place your feet flat on the floor instead of on a bench.

Advanced
Place a weight disc across your lap to increase the resistance.

THE ARMS

Lying triceps extension

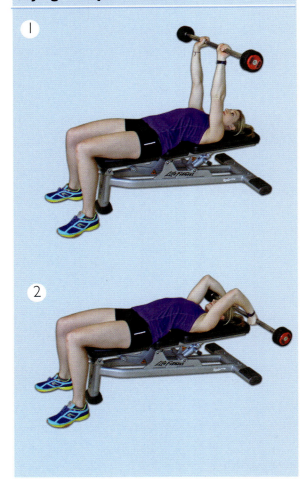

Target muscles
Triceps (especially the long inner and medial heads)

Also used: brachioradialis

Starting position
1. Lie on your back on a flat bench. If you have an excessive arch in your back, place your feet on the end of the bench or on a step.
2. Hold a barbell or EZ-bar with your hands slightly less than shoulder-width apart, palms facing forwards.
3. The bar should be positioned directly over your head with your arms fully extended.

The movement
1. Keeping your upper arms absolutely stationary, bend your elbows as you lower the bar until it just touches your forehead.
2. Hold for a count of 2, then straighten your arms back to the starting position.

Tips
- For maximum muscle development, straighten your arms fully at the end of the movement.
- Keep your elbows perfectly still – do not allow them to move out to the sides, or backwards with the bar.
- Keep your lower back firmly pressed down on the bench.
- Lower the bar as far back as you can safely to achieve the greatest ROM.

Variation
Lying dumbbell triceps extension
Use a dumbbell instead of a barbell and place your hands against the inner side of one of the end plates. You may also perform this exercise holding a pair of dumbbells, palms facing each other, or a single dumbbell, one arm at a time.

Triceps kickback

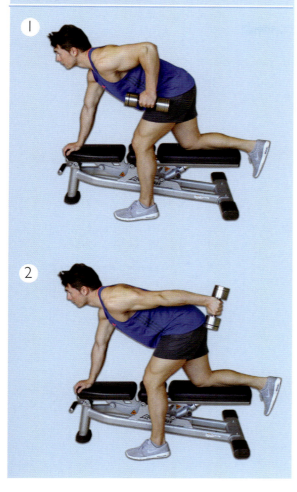

Target muscles
Triceps (especially the outer and medial heads)

Starting position
1. Hold a dumbbell in one hand.
2. Bend forwards from the waist until your torso is parallel to the floor.
3. Place your other hand and knee on a bench to stabilise yourself – your back should be flat and horizontal.
4. Bend the working arm to 90 degrees at the elbow. Bring it up so that your upper arm is parallel to, and close to, the side of your body, and the dumbbell is hanging straight down below the elbow.

The movement
1. Keeping your elbow stationary, extend your arm backwards until your arm is straight and horizontal.
2. Hold for a count of 2, then slowly return to the starting position.

Tips
- Extend your arm under control – do not swing the dumbbell back.
- Keep your upper arm fixed – only your forearm moves.
- Keep your lower back flat and still.
- Use a relatively light weight as the exercise is harder to perform than many people imagine.

Seated overhead triceps extension

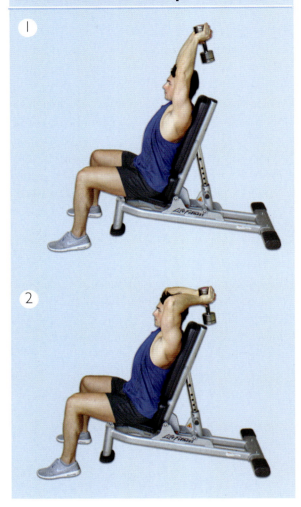

Target muscles
Triceps

Starting position
1. Sit on a bench, feet flat on the floor.
2. Grasp one end of a dumbbell with both hands, palms up, and raise it above your head, arms extended.

The movement
1. Keeping your upper arms stationary, slowly lower the dumbbell behind your head until you feel a stretch in your triceps.
2. Hold for a moment, then press the weight back up until your arms are fully extended.

Tips
- Keep your upper arms vertical so your elbows point directly overhead at all times. This will ensure the focus is kept on the triceps and does not involve the shoulders.
- Lock your elbows in the top overhead position (but make sure your arms are in a vertical line). This produces a stronger contraction of the triceps.
- Keep your torso erect throughout the movement – make sure you use a weight that isn't too heavy.

Variation
One arm overhead extension
This exercise can be done one arm at a time, holding a dumbbell in one hand.

THE ABDOMINALS

14

Well-defined abdominals are the product of hard training, careful eating and low body-fat levels. If you are after a rippling six-pack, you need to reduce your abdominal fat layer for the muscles to show through. Increasing their size alone through exercise will not be enough. For these muscles to become visible, men need to have 10–12 per cent body fat and women need to have 15–18 per cent body fat – ranges that are below those considered healthy among the general population but that are compatible with improved sports performance.

Strong abdominals help you perform virtually every strength training exercise and sports movement, and improve core stability (see p. 27). Abdominal training is also important for the prevention of lower-back injuries, since these muscles help stabilise the pelvis which, in turn, helps maintain proper spine alignment. You should add a lower-back exercise such as back extensions to your abdominal routine to help balance abdominal strength.

EXERCISES FOR THE ABDOMINALS

Crunch
Exercise ball crunch
Reverse crunch
Oblique crunch
V-sits
Medicine ball twist
Hip thrust
Side crunch
Hanging leg raise
Exercise ball pull-in
Plank
Side bridge/plank
Exercise ball jackknife/pike
Roll-out with exercise ball
Cable rotation

MUSCLE KNOW-HOW

The abdominals are comprised of four main muscle groups:

1. the rectus abdominis (the 'six-pack' muscle), running from your pubic bone to your lower ribs, which flexes the torso so the ribcage moves towards the pelvis
2. the external obliques, running diagonally from the lower ribs to the opposite hip, which bend the torso sideways and rotate it to the opposite side when flexing forwards
3. the internal obliques, running in the opposite direction to the external obliques, which help the rectus abdominis bend the torso forwards, as well as rotating it to the same side to which they are located
4. the transverse abdominis, a deep, flat sheath of muscle running across the torso, which acts as a muscular girdle to support the contents of the abdomen.

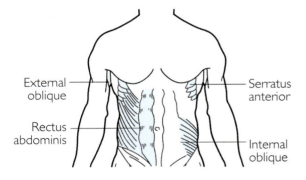

Figure 14.1 The abdominal muscles

Back strain?

Weak abdominals are often associated with back problems. This is because slack abdominal muscles can become overstretched and this, when combined with tight hip flexors (connecting the thigh bone to the lower vertebrae), can cause the pelvis to tilt forwards (lordosis), creating an excessive arch in the lower back and potential back pain. Strong abdominals support and stabilise the pelvis and lower back. Strengthening these muscles (and stretching the hip flexors) will eliminate excessive arching in the lower back, give good posture and minimise potential back problems.

Maintain a neutral alignment of the spine at all times – during everyday activities as well as when exercising – by keeping the natural 'S' contour of the spine. Your ears, shoulders, hips, knees and ankles should form a perfectly straight line when viewed from the side. This neutral position distributes the load more evenly and minimises stress to the vertebrae and discs of the spine.

TECHNIQUE TIPS

Gadgets and machines are unnecessary – you can develop great abdominals from the basic exercises that require nothing more than the floor and perhaps an exercise ball.

The secret to effective abdominal exercising is mental focus and technique. You should concentrate on each part of the movement, keeping it slow and controlled. Don't worry about how far you are moving – it's the feel that is most important. The most common error is to perform the movements too fast, aiming for a high number of repetitions. High repetitions will not work the important FT muscle fibres that give your abdominals good shape, nor will they increase definition or remove fat.

Although your spine flexes during many of the exercises, keep your neck, head and shoulders in alignment; don't press your chin into your chest – imagine you are holding an apple under your chin and keep a gap of that size at all times when performing the exercises.

The abdominals are the same as any other muscle and should be trained in the same fashion: no more than every other day and no more than 12–15 repetitions per set. So slow down, visualise your abdominals working and focus on feeling the contraction through the full ROM. When it starts to hurt (not to be confused with actual pain), take a short rest, then complete the exercise or move on to the next.

The sit-up controversy

The traditional feet-restrained sit-up is not recommended as it can put stress on the lower back and aggravate back pain. This is because the psoas – a hip flexor, which attaches to the fourth and fifth lumbar vertebrae – is involved in the movement (even if your knees are bent). When you bring your chest towards your hips from a lying position, the hip flexors initially do most of the work. Only in the last part of the movement do the abdominals contract. So, not only is the movement largely ineffective for the abs, it can also put stress on the lower back. Keep your knees slightly bent and feet unsecured to minimise hip flexor involvement when doing abdominal exercises.

Crunch

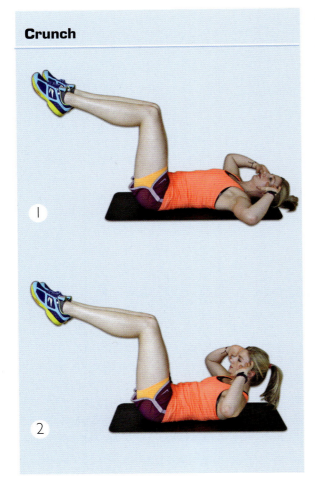

Target muscles
Rectus abdominis (mainly upper part)

Starting position
1. Lie flat on your back – on the floor or an abdominal bench – with your knees bent over your hips and your ankles touching. If you are on the floor, rest your feet on a bench with your knees bent at 90 degrees.
2. Place your hands lightly by the sides of your head or across your chest.
3. Press your lower back to the floor or bench.

The movement
1. Use your abdominal strength to raise your head and shoulders from the floor or bench. You should only come up about 10 cm and your lower back should remain on the floor or bench.
2. Hold this position for a count of 2.
3. Let your body uncurl slowly back to the starting position.

Tips
- Focus on moving your ribs towards your hips.
- Do not pull your head with your hands – keep your elbows out and relaxed.
- Exhale as you contract your abdominals.

Variations
Easier
To make the movement easier, place your feet flat on the floor, knees bent at about 60 degrees, or cross your arms over your chest.

Harder
To make the exercise harder, stretch your arms overhead, crossing your palms.

Straight leg crunch
Perform the movement with your legs straight up in the air. Now your lower abs have to work isometrically with your arms in front of you, while you curl up, reaching towards your toes.

Exercise ball crunch

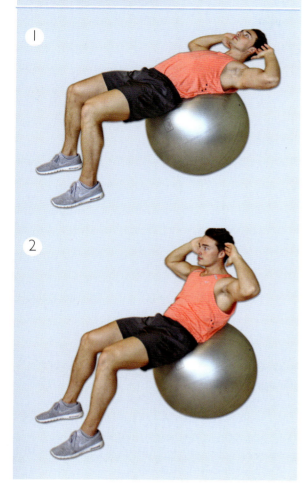

Target muscles
Rectus abdominis (mainly upper portion), transverse abdominis

Starting position
1. Sit on top of an exercise ball, feet on the floor. Slide forwards, rolling the ball under your bottom until your lower back is centred on top of the ball.
2. Cross your arms over your chest or, to make the exercise harder, place your hands by the sides of your head.

The movement
1. Making sure that you move only your upper body and that your lower back remains in contact with the ball, slowly raise your torso.
2. Hold the position for a count of 2, then lower yourself back to the starting position.

Tips
- When you lower yourself back down, keep the movement controlled.
- Do not let your upper body arch backwards or your head flop back over the ball.
- To make the movement harder, bring your body higher up on to the top of the ball.

Variation
Harder
To make the exercise harder, extend your arms behind your head. Or hold a dumbbell in front of your chest or behind your head. Make sure you start with a light weight.

Twisting exercise ball crunch
As you raise your upper body, rotate one elbow towards the opposite knee. Pause briefly then return to the starting position. Repeat to the opposite side.

Reverse crunch

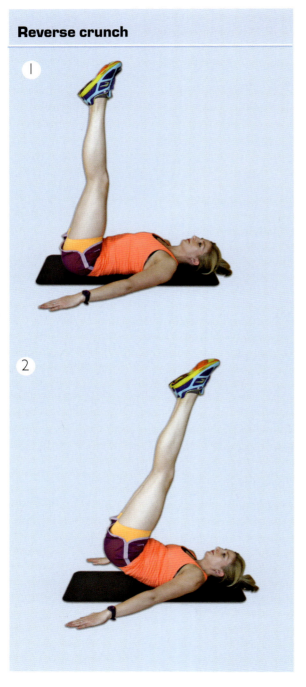

Target muscles
Rectus abdominis (mainly lower part)

Starting position
1. Lie flat on your back on the floor or on a bench with your knees bent over your hips and your ankles touching (as for crunches).
2. Place your arms on the floor alongside your body, palms flat on the floor, or hold on to the sides of the bench.
3. Press your lower back to the floor or bench.

The movement
1. Curl your hips slowly off the floor, aiming your knees towards your chest. Your hips should raise no more than 10 cm.
2. Hold for a count of 2.
3. Slowly lower your hips to the starting position, maintaining constant tension in your abdominals.

Tips
- This should be a controlled, deliberate movement. Do not jerk, swing or bounce your hips off the floor; curl up one vertebra at a time.
- Do not allow your abdominals to relax at the top of the movement or while you are uncurling.
- Exhale as you contract your abdominals.

Oblique crunch

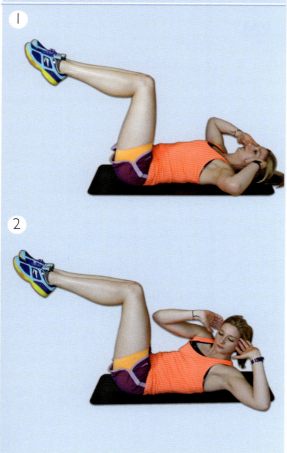

Target muscles
Internal and external obliques, rectus abdominis

Starting position
1. Lie on your back, knees bent and feet either resting on a bench or flat on the floor.
2. Place your hands by the side of your head.

The movement
1. Lift your right shoulder diagonally, aiming it towards your left knee.
2. Hold for a count of 2, then slowly return to your starting position.
3. After the required number of repetitions, complete the exercise on the other side.

Tips
- Imagine your ribcage rotating to the side as you curl up.
- Lead with your shoulder rather than your elbow.
- Make sure you lower your upper body slowly back to the floor.
- Do not twist your head, only your torso.
- Exhale as you contract your abdominals.

V-sits

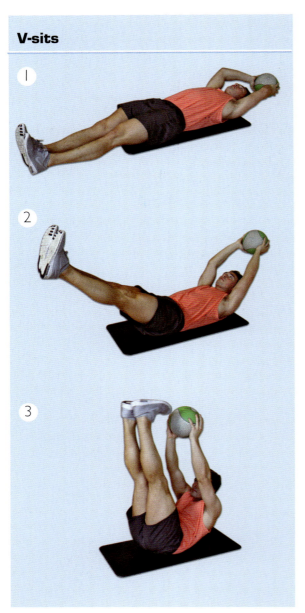

Target muscles
Rectus abdominis; transverse abdominis; obliques; hip flexors

Starting position
1. Lie flat on your back with your feet pointing straight up to the ceiling.
2. Place your hands on the floor over your head.

The movement
1. Simultaneously raise your legs and torso, reaching your hands towards your raised feet. Return to the starting position.

Tips
- Don't let your feet touch the floor.
- Use your abdominal muscles to raise your upper body off the floor, rather than swinging up to generate momentum.
- Keep your head, neck and back in a neutral position throughout the exercise.

Variations
Easier

To make the movement easier, bend your legs and extend your arms in front of you, rather than overhead.

Harder

To make the movement harder, hold a medicine ball.

Medicine ball twist

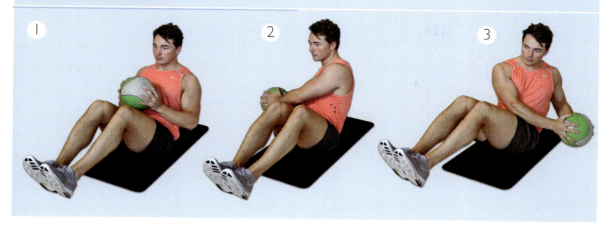

Target muscles
Internal and external obliques

Starting position
1. Sit on the floor with your knees bent and feet flat on the floor or raised off the floor.
2. Sit at about a 45 degree angle.
3. Hold a medicine ball in both hands in front of you, elbows slightly bent.

The movement
1. Twist from side to side, ensuring you initiate the movement from the waist not the shoulders, touching the ball to the floor beside you.

Tip
- To make the exercise harder, lean back further and lift your feet off the floor.

Hip thrust

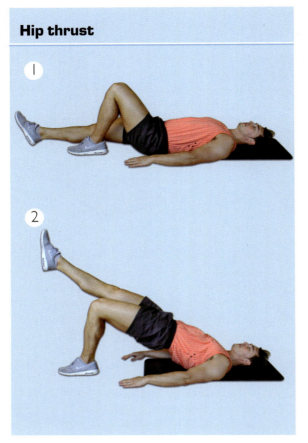

Target muscles
Rectus abdominis (mainly lower part)

Starting position
1. Lie flat on your back with your arms on the floor alongside your body, palms down.

The movement
1. Use your abs to lift your hips a few centimetres off the floor, aiming your heels towards the ceiling.
2. Hold for a count of 2.
3. Slowly lower your hips to the starting position, maintaining constant tension in your abdominals.

Tips
- Keep the movement slow and controlled – do not jerk, swing or bounce your hips off the floor.
- To make it easier, bend your knees at about 60 degrees.

Side crunch

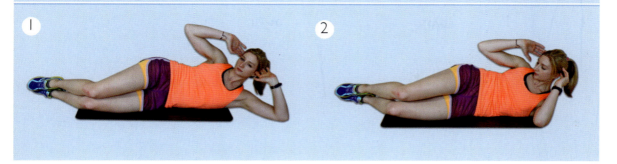

Target muscles
Internal and external obliques, rectus abdominis

Starting position
1. Lie on the floor or on an abdominal bench, on your side with your knees slightly bent.
2. Place your top arm behind your head.

The movement
1. Exhale slowly as you raise your head and shoulders a short distance off the floor or bench, aiming your ribs in the direction of your top hip.
2. Hold for a count of 2, then breathe in as you return to the starting position.
3. Repeat for the required number of repetitions, then perform the exercise on your other side.

Tips
- Aim to reduce the space between your ribs and hips.
- Do not worry if you don't reach up very far – concentrate on feeling the movement.
- Keep your head in line with your body – don't jerk it upwards.

Hanging leg raise

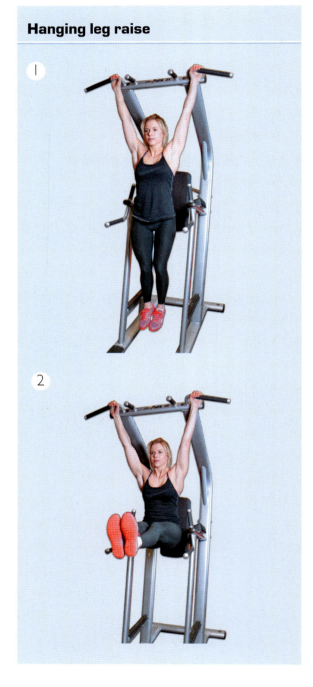

Target muscles
Rectus abdominis (especially lower portion), hip flexors

Starting position
1. Hang from a high bar with your hands shoulder-width apart. (You may use wrist or elbow straps for support.)
2. Your arms should be fully extended and your lower back slightly arched.

The movement
1. Take your legs slightly behind your body.
2. Keeping your legs almost straight, exhale and raise them upwards as high as possible. Ideally they should come just above the level of your hips. Focus on curling your hips towards your ribcage.
3. Hold for a count of 2, then slowly return your legs to the starting position.

Tips
- Do not swing your knees or use the momentum of your legs – use the strength of your abdominals to move your hips and legs.
- For maximal results, raise your legs to approximately 30–45 degrees to the horizontal. The abs shorten only when your legs go past parallel – below this, they hold a static contraction as the hip flexors raise the legs.
- To make the exercise easier, bend your knees to reduce the resistance.

Exercise ball pull-in

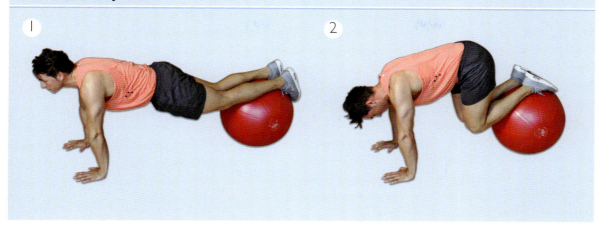

Target muscles
Rectus abdominis, transverse abdominis

Starting position
1. Get in a push-up position, placing the lower part of your shins on top of an exercise ball.
2. Your head, back, hips and knees should be in a straight line.

The movement
1. Slowly pull your knees in towards your chest, allowing the ball to roll forwards underneath your ankles.
2. Return to the starting position by straightening your legs and rolling the ball away from your body.

Tip
- Try tucking your chin into your chest during the movement.

Variation
Twisting exercise ball pull-in
Target your obliques by pulling your right knee towards your left side instead of pulling your knees in straight. Straighten, then repeat to the opposite side.

Plank

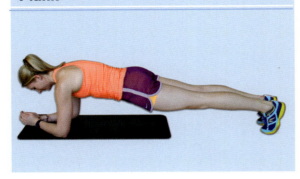

Target muscles
Rectus abdominis, transverse abdominis

Starting position
1. Lie face down on the floor with your hips and legs in contact with the floor, your upper body raised and supported on your forearms.
2. Your elbows should be directly under your shoulders by the sides of your body, palms facing down.

The movement
1. Lift your hips so that only your forearms and toes are on the floor. Keep your spine in neutral alignment – your head, back, hips and ankles should be in a straight line.
2. Hold for 60–120 seconds, then slowly lower back to the starting position.

Tips
- Keep your abs held in during the hold to protect your back.
- Check your neck, torso and legs are in a straight line.
- Make sure you don't let your bottom lift higher than your shoulders.
- Keep your shoulders pulled down and try to lengthen the distance between your shoulders and ears.

Variation
For a more advanced version, perform the plank in a push-up position, supporting your body weight on your hands instead of your forearms. Make it more challenging by raising one leg without letting the hips move. Hold, lower and repeat with the other leg.

Side bridge/plank

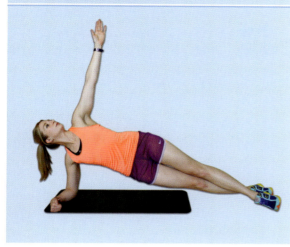

Target muscles
Obliques, transverse abdominis

Starting position
1. Lie on your right side, propping your body up on your elbow. Your elbow should be under your shoulder.
2. Your legs should be straight.

The movement
1. Lift your hips so that only your right forearm and right ankle are in contact with the floor.
2. Your body should be a straight line. Keep your spine long and in neutral alignment.
3. Hold for 5–10 seconds, then slowly lower back to the starting position. Repeat for reps, then switch sides.

Tips
- Lift your hips as high as possible without rolling forwards or back.
- Keep your hips stacked on top of each other.
- Keep your neck neutral, in line with your spine.

Variation
To make the exercise harder, support your upper body on your hand instead of your forearm. You can raise your left (top) arm to the ceiling.

Exercise ball jackknife/pike

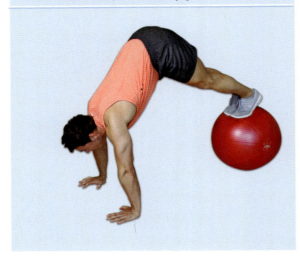

Target muscles
Obliques, transverse abdominis

Starting position
1. Get in a push-up position, resting the lower part of your shins on top of an exercise ball.
2. Make sure your arms are straight, and that your back and legs are straight.

The movement
1. Pull your lower body slowly in towards your hands, allowing the ball to roll forwards and raising your hips as high as you can.
2. Pause, contracting your abs hard, then roll the ball back to the starting position.

Tips
- This exercise requires considerable core strength and upper body strength, so practise the movement with a spotter first.
- Keep the movement smooth and controlled.
- Roll the ball in as close to your hands as possible, tucking your chin in – your torso should be almost vertical.

Roll-out (with exercise ball)

Target muscles
Obliques, transverse abdominis, rectus abdominis

Starting position
1. Kneel down in front of an exercise ball and place your hands on top of the ball, arms extended, back straight.

The movement
1. Keeping your back straight and arms extended, roll forwards as far as you can. Your head, back, hips and knees should be in a straight line.
2. Pause briefly, then pull yourself back to the starting position.

Tip
- Keep your arms extended and back straight throughout the movement.

Cable rotation

Target muscles
Obliques

Starting position
1. Grasp the handle of a shoulder-height cable pulley with both hands.
2. Step away and turn your lower body away from the pulley machine until your near arm is horizontal and straight.
3. Your feet should be a little wider than shoulder-width apart and facing away from the pulley.

The movement
1. Keeping your arms straight, rotate your torso away from the pulley until the cable makes contact with your shoulder.
2. Return to the starting position.

Tips
- Both arms should be horizontal and straight throughout the movement.
- Focus on rotating your torso rather than your hips.

BODY WEIGHT EXERCISES

15

Leg curl (on exercise ball)

Target muscles
Hamstrings
   Also used: gastrocnemius

Starting position
1. Lie on your back and place both feet on an exercise ball.
2. Place your arms next to your sides on the floor.
3. Lift your hips off the floor, forming a straight line from your feet to your neck.

The movement
1. Bend your legs, rolling the ball towards your bottom while pushing your hips up.
2. Hold this fully contracted position for a moment then slowly extend your legs back to the starting position.

Tip
- Keep your core muscles tight throughout the movement.

Single leg dead lift

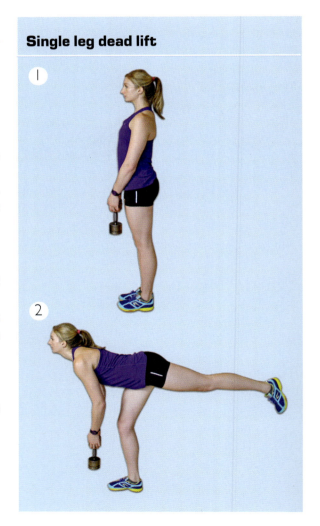

180

Target muscles
Hamstrings, gluteals

Starting position
1. Stand with your feet together and your hands just in front of your thighs.
2. Put your weight on your right leg, lifting the left foot just off the floor.

The movement
1. Hinge at your hips as you lower your torso forwards and downwards, simultaneously lifting your left leg up behind you.
2. Lower until your hands touch the floor or you feel a stretch in your hamstrings.
3. Pause briefly, then return to the starting position by raising your torso and lowering your raised leg.

Tips
- Engage your core muscles throughout the movement, keeping your tummy pulled in.
- Your feet, hips and head should all be in a straight line at the bottom of the movement.

Variations
Easier
To make the movement easier, perform the exercise standing on both legs ('double leg deadlift').

Harder
To make the movement harder, hold a kettlebell or dumbbell in your hands.

Squat (on BOSU ball)

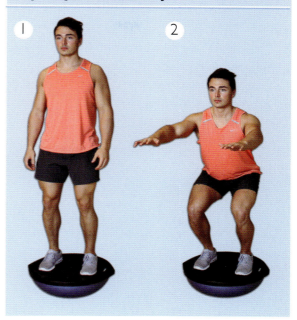

Target muscles
Gluteals, quadriceps, hamstrings, lower back, adductors, hip flexors

Starting position
1. Stand facing the BOSU ball.
2. Step on one side then slowly step on the other side. Balance your body weight on top of the BOSU.

The movement
1. Hold your arms extended in front of your body or crossed in front of your chest. Slowly lower yourself down until your thighs are parallel to the ground. Allow your hips to travel behind and keep your back straight. Keep your knees aligned over your feet, pointing in the direction of your toes.

2. Pause briefly, then straighten your legs as you return to the starting position.

Tips
- You should keep your back straight and chest high throughout the movement.
- Ensure your knees point over your toes and do not move inwards.

Single leg split squat

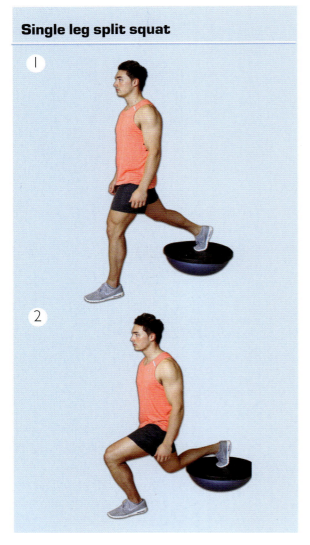

Target muscles
Quadriceps, gluteus maximus, hamstrings

Starting position
1. Stand in front of a step, BOSU ball or bench, facing away.
2. Place your rear foot on top of the elevation.

The movement
1. Drop your body downwards, bending your front knee to 90 degrees, until your rear knee is just above the floor.
2. Straighten your legs back to the starting position.

Tips
- Keep your body upright throughout the movement.
- When descending, think about dropping your hips straight down so that you avoid bending forwards.
- Keep your front knee positioned directly over your ankle – do not allow it to extend further forwards.

Lunge twist

1

2

Target muscles
Quadriceps, hamstrings, gluteals, obliques

Performing a lunge while holding and rotating a medicine ball works the muscles of the legs and core, while improving balance and proprioception.

Starting position
1. Hold a medicine ball or kettlebell in front of you with arms bent about 90 degrees.
2. Stand with your feet shoulder-width apart, toes pointing forwards. Look straight ahead.

The movement
1. Lunge forwards with your right leg, bending the knee, lowering your hips.
2. Lower yourself until your right thigh is parallel to the floor and your knee is at an angle of 90 degrees.
3. Stimultaneously twist your upper body to the right.
4. Push hard with your right leg to return to the starting position.
5. Alternate legs.

Tips
- Keep your front knee positioned directly over your ankle – do not twist at the knee.
- Keep your body erect throughout the movement.

BODY WEIGHT EXERCISES

Push-up (feet elevated)

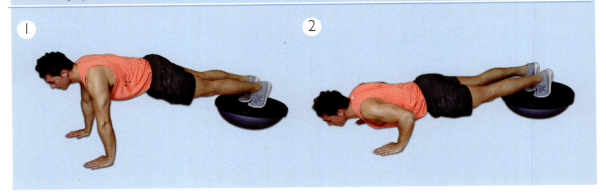

Target muscles
Pectoralis major (upper and mid chest), pectoralis minor, triceps, trunk stabilisers (transverse abdominis and the lumbar multifidus)

Starting position
1. Get in a push-up position, placing your feet on a bench, exercise ball or BOSU ball. Your head, back, hips and knees should be in a straight line (plank position).
2. Position your hands just wider than your shoulders, fingers pointing forwards.

The movement
1. Keeping your body straight, lower to the floor by bending your arms until your nose almost touches the floor. Aim your chest between your hands.
2. Straighten your arms back to the starting position. Repeat.

Tips
- Keep your spine in neutral alignment – your head, back, hips and ankles should be in a straight line – and don't let your bottom lift higher than your shoulders.
- Keep your abdominals pulled in – avoid 'swayback'.
- Keep your head in line with your spine – don't allow it to drop.

Variations
Easier
To make the movement easier, use a lower elevation or perform a standard push-up.

Harder
To make the move harder, place your feet on a higher elevation or try lifting one leg a few centimetres, keeping both legs straight.

Push-up (close grip)

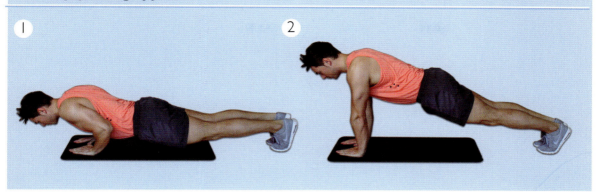

Target muscles
Pectoralis major (upper and mid chest), pectoralis minor, triceps, trunk stabilisers (transverse abdominis and the lumbar multifidus)

Starting position
1. Start in the push-up position.
2. Position your hands shoulder-width apart or narrower, fingers pointing forwards.

The movement
1. Keeping your elbows close to your body, lower your body by bending your arms so your nose almost touches the floor. Aim your chest between your hands.
2. Straighten your arms back to the starting position.

Tips
- Keep your spine in neutral alignment – your head, back, hips and ankles should be in a straight line – and don't let your bottom lift higher than your shoulders.
- Keep your abdominals pulled in – avoid 'swayback'.
- Keep your head in line with your spine – don't allow it to drop.

Variation
To make the movement easier, perform the push-ups with knees bent on the floor or placing your hands on a bench.

BODY WEIGHT EXERCISES

Side lunge

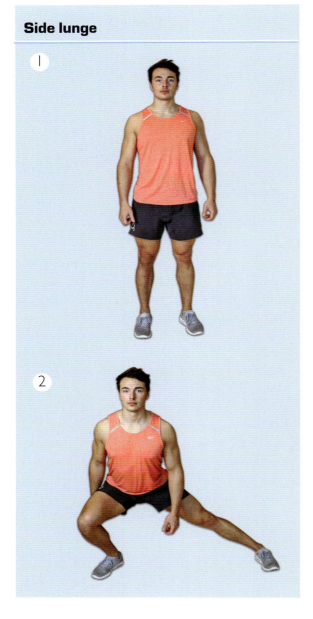

Target muscles
Gluteus maximus, quadriceps, adductors

Starting position
1. Stand with feet together, arms down by your sides.

The movement
1. Lunge to one side, placing your foot so that it points slightly outwards in the direction you are stepping. Lower your body by bending the knee of the leading leg.
2. Return to the starting position by pushing off your leading foot and straightening the leading leg.

Tips
- Keep your lead knee pointing in the same direction as your foot.
- Keep your body upright during the movement – do not lean forwards.

Variation
Make it harder by holding a pair of dumbbells by your sides.

Plank variations

Target muscles
Rectus abdominis, transverse abdominis, obliques, erector spinae

Starting position
1. Lie face down on the floor with your hips and legs in contact with the floor, your upper body raised and supported on your forearms (easier) or hands (harder).
2. Your elbows (easier) or hands (harder) should be directly under your shoulders, palms facing down.

The movement
1. Standard plank: Lift your hips so that only your forearms (easier) or hands (harder) and toes are on the floor. Keep your spine in neutral alignment – your head, back, hips and ankles should be in a straight line. This is the basic plank.
2. Plank with leg raise: Raise one leg up to the level of your shoulders. Hold for 30 seconds (or longer), then return to basic plank and lift your other leg.
3. Single arm plank: Lift one arm, extending it out in front of you.
4. BOSU plank: Using a BOSU ball (round side down), place your forearms on top of the ball.
5. Plank with rotation: Rotate your hips, shoulders and feet while raising your right arm so that you shift onto your left elbow. As you rotate, straighten your right arm up towards the ceiling. Rotate back to the starting position.

Tips
- Brace through the core and maintain proper posture throughout.
- Do not allow your hips to sag.
- Check your neck, torso and legs are in a straight line.
- Keep the shoulder blades back and together.

Variation
For a more advanced version, perform the plank in a push-up position, supporting your body weight on your hands instead of your forearms. Make it more challenging by raising one leg without letting the hips move. Hold, lower and repeat with the other leg.

Plank with leg raise
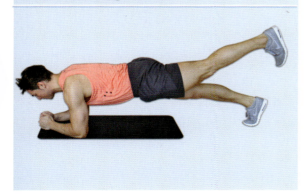

Bosu plank
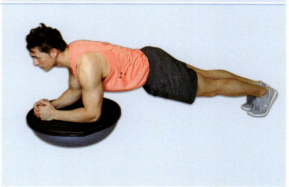

Plank with rotation

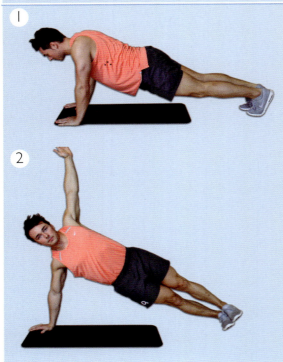

Single leg bridge

Target muscles
Hamstrings, gluteus maximus, abdominals

Starting position
1. Lie on your back with your arms by your sides, your knees bent and your feet flat on the floor.

The movement
1. Raise your hips to create a straight line from your knees to your shoulders.
2. Slowly raise and extend one leg while keeping your hips raised and level.
3. Hold for 20–30 seconds then return to the starting position and switch sides.

Tips
- Tighten your abdominals and glutes.
- Do not allow your hips to sag or drop.
- Maintain a straight line from your shoulders to your extended leg.

POWER/PLYOMETRIC EXERCISES

16

Burpees

Starting position
1. Stand with your arms by your sides.

The movement
1. Squat down, place your hands flat on the floor just in front of your feet and slightly wider than shoulder-width. Jump your feet backwards into a plank position. Immediately jump your legs back again towards your hands, performing a squat thrust.

2. Jump upwards from this squatting position, land to original standing position.

Squat jumps

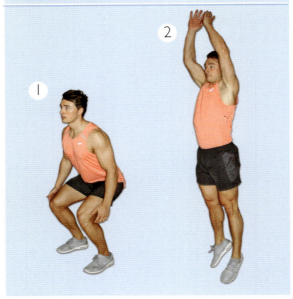

Starting position
1. Stand with your feet about shoulder-width apart, arms by your sides.

The movement
1. Squat down until your thighs are parallel to the floor and then drive up as high as possible.
2. As you land, bend your knees and sink back down into the squat position.

Tips
- As you jump upwards, push as hard as you can through the legs.
- As you land, absorb the load of the jump by landing on the front half of your feet and then transferring the weight back onto your heels as you descend into the next squat.
- Swinging your arms overhead will give you momentum.

Split squat jump

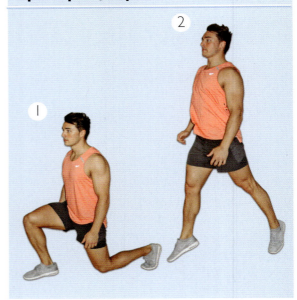

Starting position
1. Start in a split squat position with one foot forward and the other back, with both knees slightly bent.

The movement
1. Bend both knees and drive upwards off the floor, switching feet, and land with feet in opposite positions.
2. Immediately repeat the movement and continue jumps with alternating leg positions.

Tips
- Keep your torso upright throughout the movement – don't lean forwards.
- Aim to land in the same spot you jumped from.

Mountain climbers

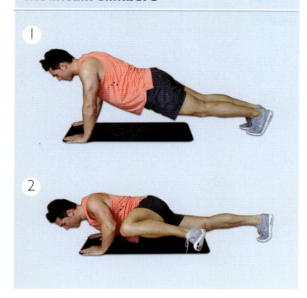

Starting position
1. Start in a straight arm plank position, with your hands slightly wider than shoulder-width.
2. Position one leg forward with your knee towards your chest and the other leg extended.

The movement
1. In a continuous movement, drive the rear leg forwards towards your chest and extend the front leg back, landing on each foot simultaneously.
2. Continue this movement with alternating leg movements.

Tips
- Keep your hips as low as possible.
- In the mid position, try to make a near-straight line from your rear foot to your head.

Plyo push-ups

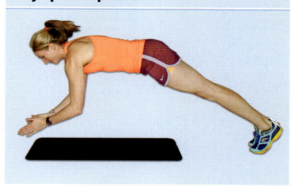

Starting position
1. Get in a push-up position – your head, hips and knees should be in a straight line (plank position) and your arms extended.

The movement
1. Bend your arms and lower your body as for a regular push-up.
2. Immediately push your upper body up hard enough for your hands to come off the floor. When they land back on the floor, go immediately into the next repetition.
3. Repeat the movement, alternating sides.

Tips
- Keep a straight line from your knees to hips to head.
- Land with your hands slightly wider than shoulder-width apart.

Variations
This movement can be performed with a medicine ball instead of a BOSU.

Make it harder by performing the exercise in a full push-up position with your feet on the floor.

Bunny hops (standing long jumps)

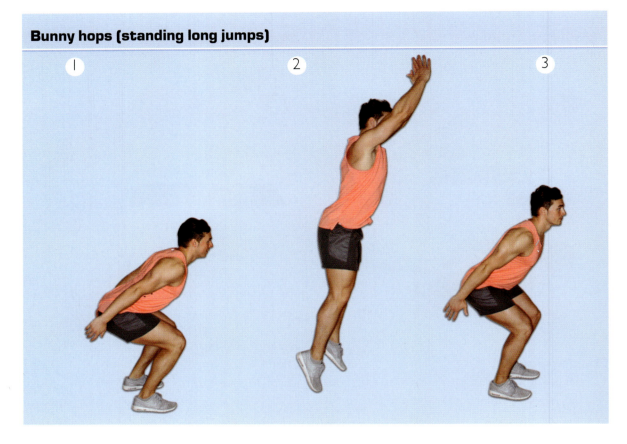

Lower body power

Starting position
1. Stand with your feet shoulder-width apart.

The movement
1. Squat down, bring both arms back behind you and jump upwards and forwards as far as possible, swinging your arms overhead.
2. Upon landing, immediately jump forward again.

Tips
- Beginners should pause and reset their position between hops. As you become accustomed to the exercise, perform two or more jumps continuously.
- Aim for a smooth sequence of drive and extension from the feet to knees to hips and arms.

Box jump (vertical jump)

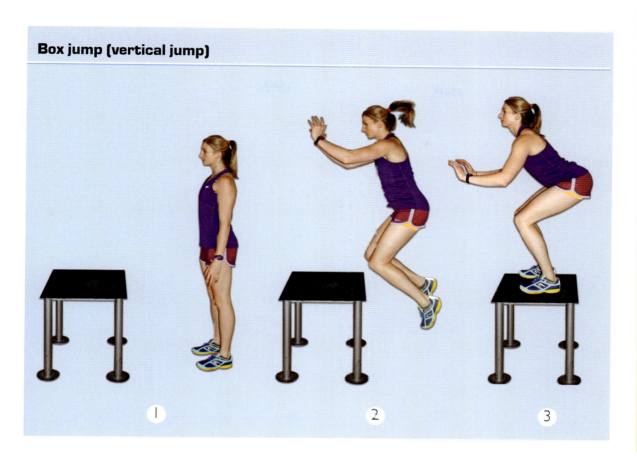

Lower body power; increases vertical jump height

Starting position
1. Stand facing a box with your feet shoulder-width apart.

The movement
1. Drop down quickly into a partial squat then extend your hips, swing your arms and push through your feet to propel yourself onto the box.
2. Land on the box, bending your knees to soften your landing.
3. Step back down and repeat.

Tip
- Use a box height that allows you to safely jump on and get both feet completely on the box (usually between 30 and 60 cm).

POWER/PLYOMETRIC EXERCISES

Vertical depth jump (jump off box)

STRENGTH TRAINING

Target muscles
Quadriceps, gluteals, hamstrings, lower body power, improves vertical leap

Starting position
1. Stand on the edge of the box with your feet shoulder-width apart.

The movement
1. Jump off the box, landing on both feet, then immediately explode upwards. Jump as high as possible.
2. Step back up on the box and repeat.

Tips
- Beginners can pause between hops. As you become accustomed to the exercise, perform two or more jumps continuously.
- Aim for a smooth sequence of drive and extension from the feet to knees to hips and arms.

Chest throw with medicine ball

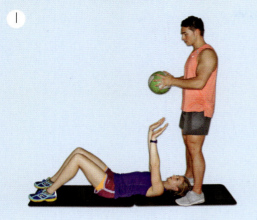
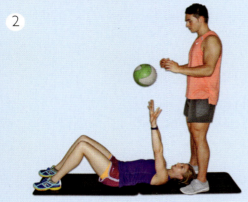
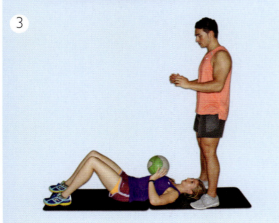

Target muscles
Chest, shoulders, triceps, upper body explosive power

Starting position
1. Lie on your back on the floor or on a bench, with your knees bent.
2. Extend your arms upwards ready to catch the ball.
3. The spotter stands just behind you, holding a medicine ball directly above your chest.

The movement
1. The spotter drops the ball above your chest.
2. Catch the medicine ball and immediately throw it forcefully upwards, extending both arms vertically.
3. The spotter catches the ball and repeats.

Tip
- Start slowly and gradually increase the speed as you get used to the exercise.

Variation
The exercise can also be performed standing. Stand facing a spotter, throwing distance apart. Throw the ball to the spotter's chest by forcefully extending both arms forwards.

Seated overhead throw

Starting position
1. Sit on the floor with your legs extended, positioned throwing distance away from a spotter.
2. Raise the medicine ball above your head with your arms bent.

The movement
1. Forcefully throw the medicine ball to the spotter.
2. Your partner catches the ball and immediately throws the ball back at you. Catch it with both hands and immediately throw it back.
3. Repeat back and forth.

Tips
• As you catch the ball, allow it to recoil behind you before throwing it back.
• Start slowly, gradually increasing the speed throughout the set.

Variation
The exercise can be performed standing instead of sitting. Stand facing your spotter, throwing distance apart. Throw the ball just above the spotter's head.

Alternatively, the throw can be performed against a wall if no partner is available.

Standing throw to floor

POWER/PLYOMETRIC EXERCISES

Target muscles
Shoulders, triceps, upper body explosive power

Starting position
1. Stand with your feet slightly wider than shoulder-width apart.
2. Raise the medicine ball above your head.

The movement
1. Bend your arms backwards a short way then throw the ball down to the floor in front of your feet.
2. As the ball bounces upwards, catch it and repeat the exercise.

Power clean

Target muscles
Total body power

Starting position
1. Stand facing a bar with the balls of your feet under the bar, shoulder-width apart.
2. Squat down, grasping the bar with an overhand grip slightly wider than shoulder-width.

The movement
1. Lift the bar from the floor by extending your hips and knees. As the bar reaches your knees, thrust your hips forwards and forcefully and quickly extend your body and move on to your toes. Then, keeping the bar close to your body, shrug your shoulders up quickly, keeping your arms straight.
2. Bend your elbows out to the sides as you begin to 'pull' your body under the bar.
3. Quickly pull your body under the bar as you rotate your arms around and under the bar. Catch the bar on your shoulders as you simultaneously bend your hips and knees into a half-squat position.
4. Stand up immediately.
5. Lower the bar by bending your hips and knees and dropping it back to the level of your thighs. Squat down with your arms straight as you lower the bar to the floor.

Tips
• Perform the exercise as one smooth continuous movement, accelerating to the highest point of the movement.
• Keep your spine in a neutral position, chest held up and eyes focused straight ahead.

Clean and jerk

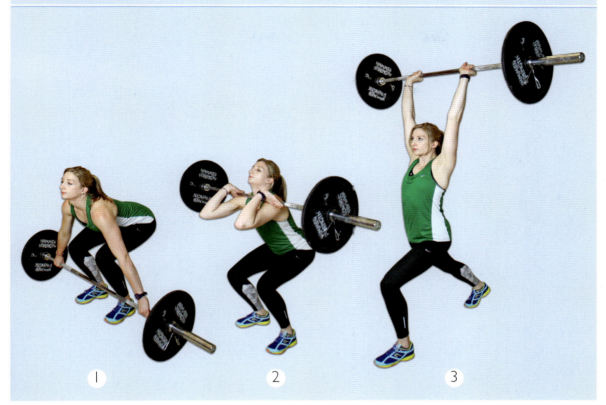

Target muscles
Total body power

Starting position
1. Stand facing a bar with the balls of your feet under the bar, shoulder-width apart.
2. Squat down, grasping the bar with an overhand grip slightly wider than shoulder-width.

The movement
1. The clean: Perform the power clean movement (p. 198).
2. The jerk: Dip your body by bending your knees slightly, then drive up through your heels. Jump one foot forwards and the other backwards, as you push the bar straight up over your head.
3. Position your feet side by side, shoulder-width apart.
4. Lower the bar back to your shoulders, then down to your thighs and finally back to the floor as you squat down.

Tips
- Perform the exercise as a two-part movement.
- Keep your spine in a neutral position, chest held up and eyes focused straight ahead.

POWER/PLYOMETRIC EXERCISES

Snatch

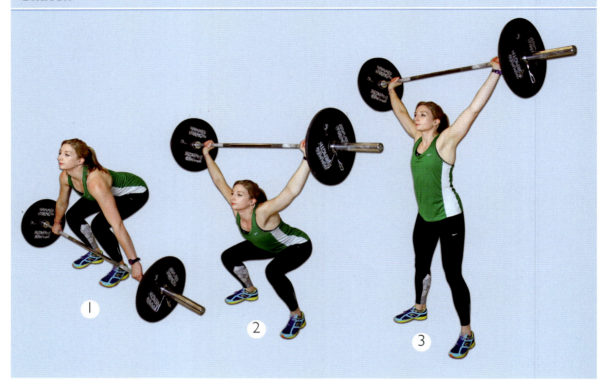

Target muscles
Total body power

Starting position
1. Stand facing a bar with the balls of your feet under the bar and shoulder-width apart.
2. Squat down, grasping the bar with an overhand grip slightly wider than shoulder-width.

The movement
1. Lift the bar from the floor by extending your hips and knees. Keep it close to your shins. As the bar passes your knees, accelerate as you extend your body and move on to your toes.
2. Then, keeping the bar close to your body, shrug your shoulders up and 'pull' yourself under the bar, sinking into a squat. As the bar passes your head, turn your wrists and push the bar straight above your head.
3. From your squatting position, stand up, straightening your legs.
4. Lower or drop the bar back to the floor under control.

Tips
- Perform as one continuous movement.
- Keep your spine in a neutral position, chest held up and eyes focused straight ahead.

THE STRETCHES

Stretching is highly beneficial for anyone involved in strength training. Not only does it provide numerous health benefits but it can also enhance your performance and muscle growth.

Flexibility

Flexibility describes the range of movement around a joint and is limited by the surrounding muscles, tendons and ligaments, as well as the anatomy of the joint.

WHY STRETCH?

The benefits of stretching include:

- reduced risk of muscle strain, joint injuries and back problems
- reduced post-exercise muscle soreness
- speedier recovery
- increased range of movement (ROM) and coordination
- greater strength gains due to greater ROM
- improved body awareness
- better physical and mental relaxation.

HOW MUSCLES STRETCH

Muscle tension is detected by receptors within the muscles and tendons, called muscle spindles. These spindles monitor changes in the muscle's length and rate of change of length. One of their jobs is to protect the muscles from injury. Stretch too far or too fast and they cause a reflex contraction to stop the movement.

Tendons – which attach muscles to bone – also contain receptors called golgi tendon organs (GTOs), which detect increases in tension and cause the muscle to relax to prevent injury. When a high force is registered, the GTOs cause the muscle to relax and the excessive tension is removed, and with it the possibility of injury. To stretch very tight muscles, you need to stimulate the GTOs rather than the muscle spindles. Slow static stretching is the best way to achieve this.

HOW STRETCHING ENHANCES MUSCLE GROWTH

Incorporating stretching into your strength training programme will result in greater muscle growth, and a lower risk of injury and muscle imbalances.

If you avoid stretching, you limit your ROM and your muscle growth potential.

Stretching helps elongate the muscle fascia, the strong protective sheath of connective tissue covering all muscles and their cells, thus allowing the muscle underneath room in which to grow. Fascia tissue can become thick and tough if the muscles are not stretched and are subjected to a limited ROM. Stretching increases flexibility, giving the muscles and joints a greater ROM. It can prevent muscle soreness and promote faster recovery between workouts, helping to release lactic acid from the muscle cells into the bloodstream so that it does not hinder further muscle contraction. Therefore, stretching during your workout may enable you to train harder and longer.

Stretching improves posture as well, and gives the body a more athletic or graceful appearance instead of that clumsy awkward gait that many bodybuilders develop.

Strength through stretching is related to your GTO threshold, which limits a contraction well short of the point at which tendons would be injured. Stretching gives the muscles the ability to contract more efficiently without shutting down in response to stretched tendons. Obviously, it is desirable to have a high GTO reflex threshold, as this allows you to lift heavier weights and do more reps without the GTOs inhibiting muscle action. The higher the GTO threshold, the more intensely you can train, and the greater the gains in size and strength. Stretching your muscles regularly can help raise your GTO threshold, some experts estimate, by up to 15–20 per cent.

STRETCHING AND MUSCLE IMBALANCE

Stretching will help you avoid injuries and muscle imbalances. Poor flexibility affects other muscles around them. Muscles work in pairs, so if one muscle is tense, this will stimulate the GTO in the opposite muscle, which will relax to accommodate this. If this tension continues, it may cause the relaxed paired muscle to become permanently inhibited and weakened. One example of this in bodybuilders is tightness in the front of the shoulders inhibiting the muscles around the rear shoulders, leading to shoulder mobility problems and pain during certain movements. Muscle imbalances can also occur around the pelvis and affect your posture, the ability to train correctly, and injury risk. Imbalances can occur through sitting at your desk all day, training with poor technique, or overtraining one muscle group (e.g. chest) without training other muscles in the body (e.g. back).

WHEN TO STRETCH?

Research suggests that static stretching before exercise has no effect on performance, injury risk or post-exercise muscle soreness. In fact, it may over-lengthen muscles and, conversely, reduce their ability to contract strongly during your workout. Instead, you should perform dynamic stretches – exaggerated movements that simulate the activity you are warming up for – before training. These may include arm circles, freestanding squats or shoulder circles.

The best time to perform static stretches is when the muscles are very warm, after a workout, or in a separate stretch session (after warming up). Stretching a cold muscle increases the risk of injury and reduces the effectiveness of the stretch.

> **Static stretching**
> This is stretching a muscle to the point of tension and holding it there. This is good for improving flexibility, and should be performed after, not before, a workout.
>
> **Dynamic stretching**
> This is moving the body through exaggerated movements similar to the workout activity without using momentum. This is good as part of a warm-up but not ideal for improving flexibility.

HOW TO STRETCH

1. Ideally, stretching should be done after a workout but can also be done during the rest intervals between sets.
2. Alternatively, stretch between workouts as a separate session, but only after a thorough warm-up (5–10 minutes of some light aerobic activity or a hot bath).
3. Perform static stretches and avoid bouncing. This is a safer method of stretching a muscle.
4. Gradually ease into position, all the time focusing on relaxing the muscle.
5. Stretch only as far as is comfortable and then hold that position. As the muscle relaxes, ease further into the stretch, gradually increasing the ROM.
6. Never hold your breath. Exhale and relax as you go into the stretch and then breathe normally.
7. Never go past the point of discomfort or pain. You could pull or tear the muscle/tendon.
8. Stretches performed at the end of a workout, or during a separate session (developmental stretching), should be held for 30 seconds or more to allow stretching in the connective tissue and muscle.
9. Release from the stretch slowly.

THE STRETCHES

Standing quadriceps stretch

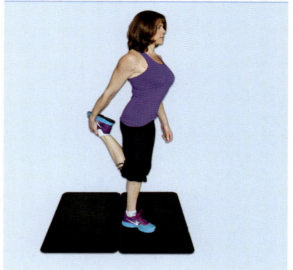

- Hold on to a sturdy support.
- Bend one leg behind you and hold the ankle.
- Keep your thighs level, knees close, keep a small gap between your heel and backside, and push your hips forwards until you feel a good stretch.
- Repeat on the other side.

Adductor stretch

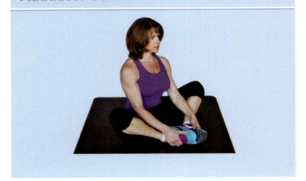

- Sit on the floor and place the soles of your feet together.
- Hold on to your ankles and press your thighs down using your elbows.
- Keep your back straight.

Hips/gluteal/outer thigh stretch

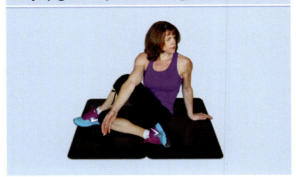

- Sit on the floor with one leg out straight and then cross your other foot over it.
- Place the elbow of the arm on the same side as your straight leg on the outside of the bent knee and slowly look over your shoulder on the side of the bent leg.
- Keep your opposite arm behind your hips for stability.
- Apply pressure to the knee with your elbow.
- Repeat on the other side.

Hip flexor stretch

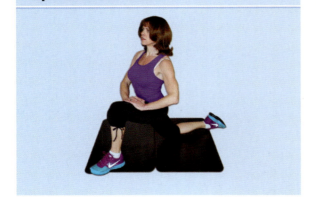

- From a kneeling position, take a large step forwards so that your knee makes a 90-degree angle and is directly over your foot.
- Keep your body upright and press your rear hip forwards, keeping it square.
- Repeat on the other side.

Lying glute stretch

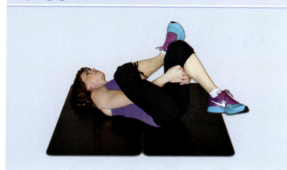

- Lie on the floor with your knees bent and feet on the floor.
- Cross the lower leg over the thigh of the other leg.
- Grasp the back of the thigh with both hands.
- Pull your leg towards your torso and hold.
- Repeat with the other leg.

Calf stretch

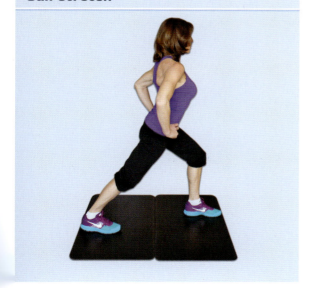

- From a standing position, take an exaggerated step forwards, keeping your rear leg straight. Use a wall for support if you wish.
- Your front knee should be at 90 degrees and positioned above your foot.
- Lean forwards slightly so that your rear leg and body make a continuous line.
- Repeat on the other side.

Lower back stretch

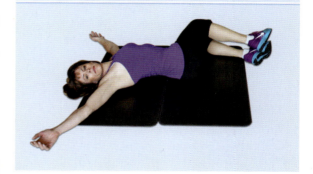

- Lie on your back, knees bent and arms straight out to the side.
- Rotate both legs to each side, keeping head, shoulders and arms in contact with the floor.

Upper back stretch

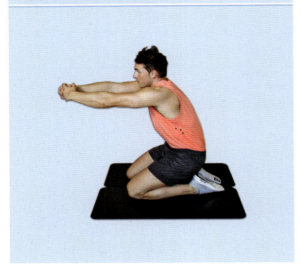

- Kneel on the floor.
- Clasp your hands together and push your arms straight out in front of you at shoulder height so you feel a good stretch between the shoulder blades.

Shoulder stretch

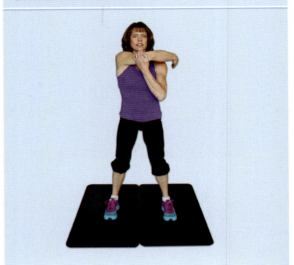

- Grab one elbow with your opposite hand.
- Gently pull it across your body, aiming the elbow towards the opposite shoulder.
- Repeat on the other side.

Chest/biceps stretch

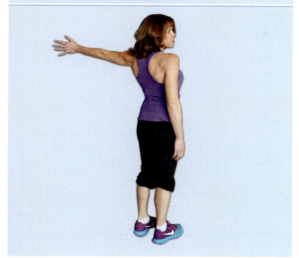

- With your arm fully extended, hold on to an upright support at shoulder level. Alternatively, you can use your training partner as support.
- Gently turn your body away from your arm, pressing your shoulder forwards.
- Repeat on the other side.

Triceps stretch

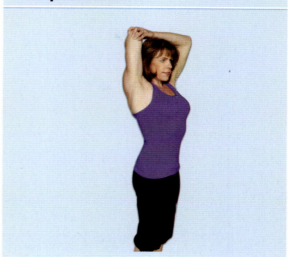

- Place one hand between your shoulder blades, hand pointing downwards and elbow pointing upwards.
- Use your opposite hand to gently press down on your elbow until you feel a stretch in the triceps.
- Repeat on the other side.

SUMMARY OF KEY POINTS

- Stretching increases flexibility and range of movement, and promotes faster recovery.
- Stretching should be performed only when the muscles are warm.
- Stretching is most beneficial when done between sets and/or after a workout.
- Ease into the stretch, hold and relax, and then gradually release.
- Avoid bouncing and any position where you feel discomfort.
- To improve flexibility, stretches should be held for a minimum of 30 seconds.

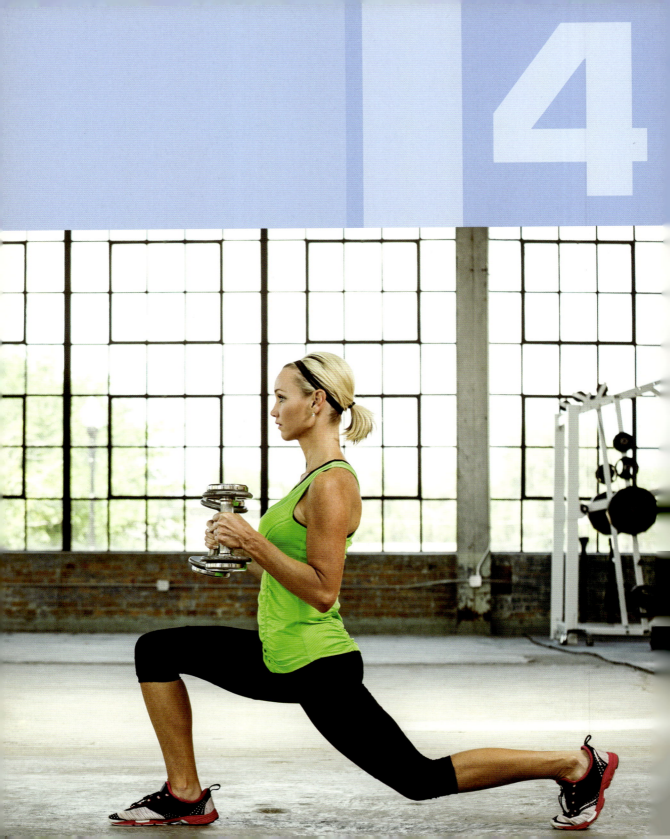

PART **FOUR**

TRAINING PROGRAMMES

Finally, here are the training programmes!

There are three basic programmes, for beginners, intermediates and advanced trainers, each designed to meet specific fitness and health goals. There are also additional programmes designed to meet different needs, for example to improve performance in different sports or to reduce the risk of injury. All the programmes draw together the scientific theory covered in Parts 1, 2 and 3. Use them as a basis for developing your own individual plan. Happy training!

THE BEGINNER'S PROGRAMME

18

This 12-week programme is designed for those with less than 6 months of strength training experience or those coming back from a lay-off of longer than 3 months.

The goal of the first 3 weeks is to introduce your muscles to the stimulus of lifting weights and familiarise you with the exercises. You'll increase your overall fitness and strength, at the same time reducing your body fat levels.

For the first 6 weeks, the introductory workout is a circuit routine because you do one set of each exercise with short rests in between. It works all the major muscle groups, and builds a good foundation of strength (or tone) and muscular endurance. The workout contains some of the most effective movements to strengthen muscles for each body part, incorporating compound exercises that work more muscle fibres through a greater diversity of angles.

From weeks 7–12, you'll use what's called a split routine. This is designed to challenge your body more. This phase should lead to noticeable increases in strength, muscle tone and muscular endurance.

You'll no longer be doing a full-body routine; the volume of work is too great to fit into one workout. Instead, you'll split your routine into two and employ the sets training method.

Workout 1 will include upper body exercises for the chest, shoulders and back, while workout 2 will include mostly lower body exercises for the legs as well as for biceps and triceps. Abdominal exercises are included in both.

Q & A

HOW MANY REPS DO I NEED TO DO?

During the first 12 weeks, you're aiming to develop muscular endurance rather than size so you should do 12–15 reps per set.

HOW MUCH WEIGHT SHOULD I USE?

Select weights that allow you to complete the prescribed number of repetitions. The last couple should feel reasonably hard. If 15 reps are easy, you need to use a heavier weight. But don't pile on so much that you're compromising technique. If you cannot complete the set or you feel an intense burn in your muscles, you need to select a lighter weight. To be safe, choose a weight lighter than you think you can do and go from there.

HOW SLOWLY DO I NEED TO GO?

Count 2 seconds up, 3 seconds down. Lifting weights too fast lets momentum, gravity and other muscles help out, preventing the target muscles from getting the full benefit. The lowering (eccentric) phase of the lift is just as important for building strength and size as the raising (concentric) phase.

HOW MANY SETS SHOULD I DO?

For the first 6 weeks, you do a single set of each exercise before moving on to the next one. Thereafter, in order to continue making gains in strength, you have to step up the workout intensity. Doing 3 sets of each exercise increases the workload for each body part and is considered effective for maximum development of strength and size.

HOW LONG SHOULD I REST BETWEEN WORKOUTS?

Rest at least 48 hours before training the same muscle group again. Muscles need time to repair and rebuild themselves. They don't grow during your workout – they rebuild in between workouts, at rest. During the first 6 weeks, when you will be doing a whole-body routine, schedule your workouts every other day – Monday, Wednesday and Friday, for example – to give your muscles time to recuperate. During the second 6 weeks, when you will be doing a split routine, leave at least 48 hours between training the same body part – do workout 1 on Monday and Thursday, and workout 2 on Tuesday and Friday, for example.

WARM UP AND COOL DOWN

Always warm up with 5–10 minutes cardiovascular exercise before your workout to reduce your risk of injury. After completing your workout, spend 5 minutes stretching.

BEGINNER'S WORKOUT: WEEKS 1–3

- Complete the following workout twice a week for the first week. If you feel comfortable, increase this to 3 times a week for the following 2 weeks.
- Rest for at least 1 day between workouts.
- Do one circuit for the first week.
- Step up to 2 circuits in weeks 2 and 3, taking 2–3 minutes' rest in between.
- Move between exercises with minimum rest.
- You should complete the workout in well under 30 minutes.

Table 18.1	Beginner's workout: weeks 1–3	Week 1		Weeks 2–3	
Body part	Exercise	Circuits	Reps	Circuits	Reps
Warm up with a 5-minute cardiovascular activity and some mobility movements					
Legs	Leg press	1	15	2	15
Chest	Vertical bench press machine	1	15	2	15
Upper back	Machine row	1	15	2	15
Shoulders	Overhead press machine	1	15	2	15
Biceps	Dumbbell curl	1	15	2	15
Triceps	Triceps push-down	1	15	2	15
Lower back	Back extension (on floor)	1	15	2	15
Abdominals	Crunch	1	15	2	15
Calves	Standing calf raise	1	15	2	15

BEGINNER'S WORKOUT: WEEKS 4-6

- Complete the following workout 3 times a week.
- Rest for at least 1 day between workouts.
- Move between exercises with minimum rest.
- Do 2–3 circuits with 2–3 minutes' rest between them.
- You should complete the workout in less than 40 minutes.
- Make sure your technique is sound before increasing the weights.

Concentrate on using a complete range of movement and perfecting your training technique. Don't be tempted to add more sets or push heavy weights. You need to give your body sufficient time to adjust to this type of training. Pushing yourself too hard will not produce greater benefits – recovery times will be lengthened and you may end up overtraining and risking injury.

Table 18.2	Beginner's workout: weeks 4–6		
Body part	**Exercise**	**Circuits**	**Reps**
Warm up with a 5-minute cardiovascular activity and some mobility movements			
Legs	Leg press	2	15
Hamstrings	Seated leg curl	2	15
Chest	Bench press machine	2	15
Chest	Pec-deck flye	2	15
Upper back	Machine row	2	15
Upper back	Lat pull-down	2	15
Shoulders	Overhead press machine	2	15
Shoulders	Dumbbell lateral raise	2	15
Biceps	Dumbbell curl	2	15
Triceps	Triceps push-down	2	15
Lower back	Back extension (on floor or ball)	2	15
Abdominals	Crunch	2	15
Calves	Standing calf raise	2	15

BEGINNER'S WORKOUT: WEEKS 7–9

- Complete 3 workouts per week, alternating workout 1 and workout 2, e.g. workout 1 on Monday and Friday; workout 2 on Wednesday.
- Do 3 sets of 12 reps of 2 exercises for chest, upper back and shoulders.
- Do 1 set of 12 reps for lower back, abdominals, biceps, triceps and calves.
- Rest 30–45 seconds between sets of the same exercise; rest for approximately 60–90 seconds between different exercises.
- Use a heavier weight but maintain form.

Table 18.3	Beginner's workout: weeks 7–9 (workout 1)		
Body part	**Exercise**	**Sets**	**Reps**
Warm up with a 5-minute cardiovascular activity and some mobility movements			
Chest	Dumbbell press	3	12
Chest	Pec-deck flye	3	12
Upper back	Pull-up/chin-up machine	3	12
Upper back	Lat pull-down to front	3	12
Shoulders	Dumbbell press	3	12
Shoulders	Dumbbell lateral raise	3	12
Lower back	Back extension with exercise ball	1	12
Abdominals	Exercise-ball crunch	1	12
	Reverse crunch	1	12
	Plank	1	Hold for 30 seconds

Table 18.4 Beginner's workout: weeks 7–9 (workout 2)

Body part	Exercise	Sets	Reps
Warm up with a 5-minute cardiovascular activity and some mobility movements			
Legs	Split squat	3	12
Hamstrings	Seated leg curl	3	12
Quads	Leg extension	3	12
Calves	Standing calf raise	3	12
Biceps	Barbell curl	1	12
Triceps	Bench dip	1	12
Abdominals	Oblique crunch	1	12
	V-sits	1	12
	Medicine ball twist	1	12

Table 18.5 Beginner's workout: weeks 10–12 (workout 1)

Body part	Exercise	Sets	Reps
Warm up with a 5-minute cardiovascular activity and some mobility movements			
Chest	**Choose 3 exercises:** Bench press (machine or barbell) Incline dumbbell press Pec-deck flye Dumbbell flye	2	12
Upper back	**Choose 3 exercises:** Machine row Lat pull-down to front Seated cable row One arm dumbbell row	2	12
Shoulders	**Choose 2 exercises:** Overhead press machine Dumbbell lateral raise Dumbbell press	2	12
Lower back	Back extension on floor/bench/ball	3	12
Abdominals	Crunch (on floor or exercise ball) Oblique crunch Reverse crunch	2	12

BEGINNER'S WORKOUT: WEEKS 10–12

- Complete 3 workouts per week, alternating workout 1 and workout 2.
- Rest 30–45 seconds between sets of the same exercise; rest for approximately 60–90 seconds between different exercises.
- Do 2 sets of 3 exercises for legs, chest and upper back.
- Do 2 sets of 2 exercises for shoulders, biceps, triceps, calves and abdominals.

Table 18.6	Beginner's workout: weeks 10–12 (workout 2)		
Body part	**Exercise**	**Sets**	**Reps**
Warm up with a 5-minute cardiovascular activity and some mobility movements			
Legs	**Choose 3 exercises:** Leg press machine Front lunge Split squat Seated leg curl Leg extension Dumbbell step-ups	2	12
Calves	**Choose 2 exercises:** Dumbbell single leg calf raise Standing calf raise	2	12
Biceps	**Choose 2 exercises:** Dumbbell curl Barbell curl Cable curl	2	12
Triceps	**Choose 2 exercises:** Triceps push-down Bench dips Lying triceps extension	2	12
Abdominals	**Choose 2 exercises:** Plank Side bridge (plank) Hip thrust	2	12

THE INTERMEDIATE'S PROGRAMME

19

This 6-month programme is for trainers who have either completed the 12-week beginner's programme or have been training consistently for at least 6 months.

This programme is designed to increase muscle size and strength, and should be followed for a minimum of 6 months before progressing to the advanced programme (see p. 223). It includes new exercises to stimulate continued muscle development and a different split routine. The goal is to challenge your body further by working with greater intensity and including more volume.

You'll be training your body over three different workouts instead of two as you did in the final 6 weeks of the beginner's programme. Workout 1 trains chest, upper back and abdominals. Workout 2 trains shoulders, biceps, triceps and abdominals, and workout 3 trains legs, abdominals and lower back. By splitting your body into three parts you can train with even greater intensity and include more volume.

Q & A

HOW MANY REPS DO I NEED TO DO?

The number of exercises and sets per body part is increased and you'll now be working in the rep range of 8–12. For muscle size and strength, you should do 8–12 reps per set with 60–90 seconds' rest in between sets. The pyramid training method is used in this programme, so the weight increases and the repetitions decrease progressively with each set (see p. 24).

HOW MUCH WEIGHT SHOULD I USE?

Choose a weight that will make the last 1 or 2 reps challenging. If you can complete 12 reps easily, you need to use a heavier weight. Only increase the weight when you are ready, adding 2.5–5 kg so that you're able to lift only within the 8–12 rep range again.

HOW SLOWLY DO I NEED TO GO?

Count 2 seconds up, 3 seconds down. Lifting weights too fast lets momentum, gravity and other muscles help out, preventing the target muscles from getting the full benefit. The lowering (eccentric) phase of the lift is just as important for building strength and size as the raising (concentric) phase.

HOW MANY SETS SHOULD I DO?
Do 3 sets of each exercise, although sometimes going above or below this (2–6 sets) will produce similar benefits. You'll notice now that as intensity and volume are increased, frequency is gradually decreased. These are important components of a well-designed programme.

HOW LONG SHOULD I REST BETWEEN WORKOUTS?
Now the volume and intensity has been increased, you'll need more recovery time so you should train each body part only once a week. You could train on Monday, Wednesday and Friday but, if this doesn't suit you, you could choose different days.

You have more leeway as to when you train with a three-way training split. While you're doing workout 2, for example, the muscles trained in workout 1 are getting a rest.

WARM UP AND COOL DOWN
Always warm up with 5–10 minutes cardiovascular exercise before your workout to reduce your risk of injury. After completing your workout, spend 5 minutes stretching.

Here are two workout programmes, A and B. Follow each for 1 month (4 weeks) then repeat twice so you will have completed the intermediate's programme in 6 months. The workouts include different exercises, so will keep your body challenged.

INTERMEDIATE'S WORKOUT A

- Complete each workout once a week.
- Rest 60–90 seconds between sets and 1–2 minutes between exercises.
- Most sets should fall within 8–12 reps.
- The last repetition of each set should feel extremely hard, and you should be unable to complete another one in proper form.
- Maintain strict form for each repetition, using the complete ROM.

Table 19.1	Intermediate's workout A: workout 1 (chest, upper back, abdominals)		
Body part	**Exercise**	**Sets**	**Reps**
Warm up with a 5-minute cardiovascular activity and some mobility movements			
Chest	Bench press (barbell)	3	8–12
	Incline dumbbell press	3	8–12
	Cable cross-over	2	8–12
Upper back	One arm dumbbell row	3	8–12
	Lat pull-down to front	3	8–12
	Seated cable row	2	8–12
Abdominals	Reverse crunch*	3	12–15
	Crunch*	3	12–15

* Perform as a superset – do the first exercise immediately followed by the second exercise. Rest for 1–2 minutes before repeating the superset.

Table 19.2	Intermediate's workout A: workout 2 (shoulders, arms, abdominals)		
Body part	**Exercise**	**Sets**	**Reps**
Warm up with a 5-minute cardiovascular activity and some mobility movements			
Shoulders	Shoulder press (dumbbell or barbell)	3	8–12
	Lateral raise	3	8–12
	Bent-over lateral raise	2	8–12
Biceps	Barbell curl	2	8–12
	Concentration curl	2	8–12
Triceps	Triceps push-down	2	8–12
	Lying triceps extension	2	8–12
Abdominals	Oblique crunch*	2	12–15
	Plank*	2	Hold for 60–120 seconds
	Medicine ball twist	2	12–15

* Perform as a superset – do the first exercise immediately followed by the second exercise. Rest for 1–2 minutes before repeating the superset.

Table 19.3	Intermediate's workout A: workout 3 (legs, abdominals, lower back)		
Body part	**Exercise**	**Sets**	**Reps**
Warm up with a 5-minute cardiovascular activity and some mobility movements			
Legs	Squat	3	8–12
	Split squat	3	8–12
	Leg extension	2	8–12
	Seated leg curl	2	8–12
Calves	Standing calf raise	3	12–15
Abdominals	Exercise ball pull-in*	2	12–15
	Side bridge*	2	5**
	Roll-out with ball	2	12–15
Lower back	Back extension with exercise ball	3	12–15

* Perform as a superset – do the first exercise immediately followed by the second exercise. Rest for 1–2 minutes before repeating the superset.
** Hold for 5 seconds, repeat for 5 reps on each side.

INTERMEDIATE'S WORKOUT B

- Complete each workout once a week.
- Rest 60–90 seconds between sets and 1–2 minutes between exercises.
- Most sets should fall within 8–12 reps.
- The last repetition of each set should feel extremely hard, and you should be unable to complete another one in proper form.
- Maintain strict form for each repetition, using the complete ROM.

Table 19.4	Intermediate's workout B: workout 1 (chest, upper back, abdominals)		
Body part	**Exercise**	**Sets**	**Reps**
Warm up with a 5-minute cardiovascular activity and some mobility movements			
Chest	Dumbbell press	3	8–12
	Incline dumbbell flye	3	8–12
	Push-up (feet elevated)	2	8–12
Upper back	Pull-up (or chin-up)	3	8–12
	Dumbbell pull-over	3	8–12
	Dumbbell shrug	2	8–12
Abdominals	Exercise ball crunch*	3	12–15
	Side crunch*	3	12–15

* Perform as a superset – do the first exercise immediately followed by the second exercise. Rest for 1–2 minutes before repeating the superset.

Table 19.5	Intermediate's workout B: workout 2 (shoulders, arms, abdominals)		
Body part	**Exercise**	**Sets**	**Reps**
Warm up with a 5-minute cardiovascular activity and some mobility movements			
Shoulders	Overhead press machine	3	8–12
	Upright row	3	8–12
	Bent-over lateral raise	2	8–12
Biceps	Preacher curl	2	8–12
	Incline dumbbell curl	2	8–12
Triceps	Bench dip	2	8–12
	Triceps kickback	2	8–12
Abdominals	Crunch*	3	12–15
	Medicine ball twist*	3	12–15

* Perform as a superset – do the first exercise immediately followed by the second exercise. Rest for 1–2 minutes before repeating the superset.

Table 19.6	Intermediate's workout B: workout 3 (legs, abdominals, lower back)		
Body part	**Exercise**	**Sets**	**Reps**
Warm up with a 5-minute cardiovascular activity and some mobility movements			
Legs	Leg press	3	8–12
	Front lunge	2	8–12
	Reverse lunge	2	8–12
Calves	Standing calf raise (Smith machine)	3	12–15
Abdominals	Reverse crunch*	3	12–15
	Hip thrust*	3	12–15
Lower back	Back extension (on the bench)	3	12–15

* Perform as a superset – do the first exercise immediately followed by the second exercise. Rest for 1–2 minutes before repeating the superset.

THE ADVANCED PROGRAMME

This advanced programme is a progression of the intermediate's programme. It provides a more serious workout for trainers who have completed the intermediate's programme, have trained consistently for at least a year, and are looking to add a greater variety of exercises and training techniques to their workouts.

The goal is to overload your muscles further to increase muscle strength and size. Thus it provides a higher-intensity workout. This programme is based on a similar three-way split workout to the intermediate workout but incorporates advanced training techniques – descending sets, supersets and pre-exhaustion – alongside the established basic methods of sets and pyramid training.

You can include an advanced technique once a week or once every 2 weeks. However, as they are very intense, you should avoid using these techniques too frequently on any one body part as they impose considerable stress on the muscles.

Q & A

HOW OFTEN SHOULD I DO AN ADVANCED WORKOUT?

Choose one of the following advanced workouts in place of your regular (intermediate) workout (see the periodisation chart on p. 34) once every 2 weeks. Do not use an advanced training technique on the same body part more frequently than once a fortnight otherwise you risk overtraining.

HOW MUCH WEIGHT SHOULD I USE?

Choose a weight that will make the last 1 or 2 reps challenging. If you can complete 12 reps easily, you need to use a heavier weight. Only increase the weight when you are ready, adding 2.5–5 kg so that you're able to lift only within the 8–12 rep range again.

HOW SLOWLY DO I NEED TO GO?

Count 2 seconds up, 3 seconds down. Lifting weights too fast lets momentum, gravity and other muscles help out, preventing the target muscles from getting the full benefit. The lowering (eccentric) phase of the lift is just as important for building strength and size as the raising (concentric) phase.

HOW MANY SETS SHOULD I DO?

You should do approximately 8 sets for legs, upper back, chest and shoulders, and 4 sets for biceps, triceps, calves and lower back.

HOW LONG SHOULD I REST BETWEEN WORKOUTS?

Each body part should be trained just once a week to allow sufficient recovery time between workouts. Ideally, you should train on non-consecutive days, but with a three-way training split you have some leeway – the muscles trained in the previous workout are getting a rest while you perform your next workout.

WARM UP AND COOL DOWN

Always warm up with 5–10 minutes cardiovascular exercise before your workout to reduce your risk of injury. After completing your workout, spend 5 minutes stretching.

DESCENDING SETS

Complete the first 2 sets of the exercise, performing 8–12 reps per set, then do a descending set for your last set. Complete 8–12 reps in good form, then reduce the weight by 20–30 per cent and immediately complete as many repetitions as possible until you reach 'failure'. You should be able to complete an additional 4–8 reps. If you wish, you can reduce the weight a further 20–30 per cent and complete as many reps as you can. Take 2–3 minutes' rest between sets and between exercises.

Table 20.1	Advanced workout I with descending sets (chest, arms)		
Body part	**Exercise**	**Sets**	**Reps**
Warm up with a 5-minute cardiovascular activity and some mobility movements			
Chest	Bench press (barbell or dumbbell)	3	8–12
	Incline bench press (barbell or dumbbell)	3	8–12 3rd set descending set
	Dumbbell flye (flat or incline)	2	8–12 2nd set descending set
Biceps	Dumbbell curl	2	8–12 2nd set descending set
	Concentration curl	2	8–12
Triceps	Lying triceps extension	2	8–12 2nd set descending set
	Reverse-grip triceps press-down	2	8–12
Abdominals	Oblique crunch*	2	12–15
	Hanging leg raise*	2	12–15

* Perform as a superset – do the first exercise immediately followed by the second exercise. Rest for 1–2 minutes before repeating the superset.

Table 20.2 — Advanced workout 2 with descending sets (shoulders, back)

Body part	Exercise	Sets	Reps
Warm up with a 5-minute cardiovascular activity and some mobility movements			
Shoulders	Dumbbell press	3	8–12
	Dumbbell lateral raise	3	8–12 3rd set descending set
	Upright row	2	8–12 2nd set descending set
Upper back	Barbell row	3	8–12 3rd set descending set
	Pull-up/chin-up	3	8–12 3rd set descending set
	Straight arm pull-down	2	8–12
Abdominals	Exercise ball crunch*	2	12–15
	Hip thrust*	2	12–15

* Perform as a superset – do the first exercise immediately followed by the second exercise. Rest for 1–2 minutes before repeating the superset.

Table 20.3 — Advanced workout 3 with descending sets (legs)

Body part	Exercise	Sets	Reps
Warm up with a 5-minute cardiovascular activity and some mobility movements			
Quadriceps/gluteals	Squat	3	8–12
Quadriceps	Leg extension	3	8–12 3rd set descending set
Hamstrings	Straight leg dead lift	3	8–12 3rd set descending set
Calves	Standing calf raise	3	8–12 3rd set descending set
Abdominals	Exercise ball pull-in*	2	12–15
	Side bridge*	2	5**

* Perform as a superset – do the first exercise immediately followed by the second exercise. Rest for 1–2 minutes before repeating the superset.
** Hold for 5 seconds, repeat 5 times on each side.

SUPERSETS

Pair exercises are mirror images of each other, like leg extensions and leg curls. Do the first exercise of the superset first (e.g. barbell bent-over row), followed immediately by the second superset. Rest for 1–2 minutes then repeat the process. Once you complete the prescribed number of supersets, rest for 2 minutes then move on to the next superset.

Table 20.4	Advanced workout 1 with supersets (chest, back, shoulders)		
Body part	**Exercise**	**Sets**	**Reps**
Warm up with a 5-minute cardiovascular activity and some mobility movements			
Superset No. 1			
Back	Barbell bent-over row	3	8–12
Chest	Bench press		8–12
Superset No. 2			
Back	Lat pull-down	3	8–12
Chest	Incline dumbbell press		8–12
Superset No. 3			
Shoulders	Dumbbell press	3	8–12
Trapezius	Upright row		8–12
Superset No. 4			
Shoulders	Lateral raise	3	8–12
Trapezius	Dumbbell shrug		8–12

Table 20.5	**Advanced workout 2 with supersets (quadriceps, hamstrings and calves/forearms)**		
Body part	**Exercise**	**Sets**	**Reps**
Warm up with a 5-minute cardiovascular activity and some mobility movements			
Superset No. 1			
Quadriceps	Squat	3	8–12
Hamstrings	Straight leg dead lift		8–12
Superset No. 2			
Quadriceps	Leg extension	3	8–12
Hamstrings	Seated leg curl		8–12
Superset No. 3			
Calves	Standing calf raise	3	8–12
Abdominals	Plank		Hold for 60–120 seconds

Table 20.6	**Advanced workout 3 with supersets (biceps/triceps and abdominals/lower back)**		
Body part	**Exercise**	**Sets**	**Reps**
Warm up with a 5-minute cardiovascular activity and some mobility movements			
Superset No. 1			
Biceps	Barbell curl	3	8–12
Triceps	Triceps push-down		8–12
Superset No. 2			
Biceps	Preacher curl	3	8–12
Triceps	Bench dip		8–12
Superset No. 3			
Abdominals	V-sits	3	15–20
Lower back	Superman		15–20
Superset No. 4			
Abdominals	Reverse crunch	3	15–20
Lower back	Back extension on machine		15–20

PRE-EXHAUSTION

The pre-exhaustion training method is used for chest, shoulders and legs. An isolation exercise is performed followed by a compound exercise. Rest 60–90 seconds between sets and 2–3 minutes between exercises.

Table 20.7	Day 1: advanced workout 1 with pre-exhaustion (chest, back, shoulders)		
Body part	**Exercise**	**Sets**	**Reps**
Warm up with a 5-minute cardiovascular activity and some mobility movements			
Chest	Dumbbell flye	4	8–12
	Bench press (barbell or dumbbell)	4	8–12
Shoulders	Front lateral raise	4	8–12
	Dumbbell press/overhead press machine	4	8–12
Abdominals	Exercise ball pull-in*	3	12–15
	Side bridge*	3	5**

* Perform as a superset – do the first exercise immediately followed by the second exercise. Rest for 1–2 minutes before repeating the superset.
** Hold for 5 seconds, repeat for 5 reps on each side.

Table 20.8	Day 2: advanced workout 2 with pre-exhaustion (legs)		
Body part	**Exercise**	**Sets**	**Reps**
Warm up with a 5-minute cardiovascular activity and some mobility movements			
Quadriceps	Leg extension	3	8–12
Hamstrings	Lying leg curl	3	8–12
Quadriceps/hamstrings, gluteals	Leg press	4	8–12
Calves	Standing calf raise	3	8–12
Abdominals	Roll-out with ball*	3	12–15
	Exercise ball jackknife/pike*	3	12–15

* Perform as a superset – do the first exercise immediately followed by the second exercise. Rest for 1–2 minutes before repeating the superset.

Table 20.9	Day 3: advanced workout 3 with pre-exhaustion (upper back, biceps, triceps)		
Body part	**Exercise**	**Sets**	**Reps**
Warm up with a 5-minute cardiovascular activity and some mobility movements			
Upper back	Lat pull-down	3	8–12
	Seated row	3	8–12
	Dumbbell shrug	2	8–12
Biceps	Barbell curl	2	8–12
	Concentration curl	2	8–12
Triceps	Lying triceps extension	2	8–12
	Triceps push-down	2	8–12
Abdominals	Oblique crunch*	3	12–15
	Plank*	3	Hold for 60–120 seconds
Lower back	Back extension (on floor)	3	12–15

* Perform as a superset – do the first exercise immediately followed by the second exercise. Rest for 1–2 minutes before repeating the superset.

THE ADVANCED PROGRAMME

THE STRENGTH PROGRAMME

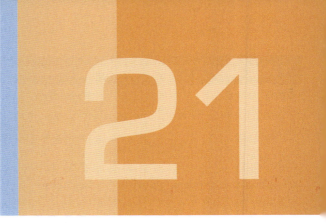

The aim of this programme is to increase pure strength. In addition to power lifters, anyone training for muscle size would benefit from including a maximum-strength phase in their training cycle (see the section on periodisation, p. 30). It can help you get through a sticking point by allowing you to lift more weight and further increase your muscle size when you resume your regular routine. The idea is that by varying the intensity, you alter the recruitment of muscle fibres so that, over time, you gain more fibres.

Training for strength involves using basic compound exercises – squats, dead lifts and bench presses – with heavy weights and low reps. This type of training causes maximum stimulation of the powerful FT muscle fibres and hence greater muscle strength. It not only increases muscle strength, but also improves joint stability and muscle mass.

Q & A

HOW LONG CAN I FOLLOW THIS WORKOUT?

You can incorporate this strength programme into your bodybuilding programme for a period of 4–6 weeks, in place of your normal workouts. After this, return to your normal routine.

HOW OFTEN SHOULD I TRAIN?

Do the workout twice a week.

HOW MUCH WEIGHT SHOULD I USE?

Using near-maximal weights – at least 85 per cent 1RM – develops maximum strength. If you do not know your 1RM, find a weight that you can just lift for 6 strict repetitions. This will approximate to 70–80 per cent 1RM. As with any bodybuilding programme, you need to increase the weight you lift gradually over time.

ANY PRECAUTIONS?

It is important to warm up thoroughly, otherwise you risk injury. Perform 5 minutes of a cardio-vascular activity followed by 2 or 3 sets of that exercise using very light weights for about 15 reps before embarking on the heavy sets. Ensure that you use the full ROM for each exercise and train using perfect technique.

HOW MANY SETS AND REPS?

Following your warm-up sets, perform 4 working sets of each exercise. Begin with weights equal to 70–80 per cent of your 1RM and do 6–8 reps. Progress to 80–90 per cent of your 1RM for 3–4 reps. You should also allow longer rest periods between sets (3–4 minutes) than in the bodybuilding programme to allow full recovery of your fuel system.

Table 21.1	Strength workout 1 (legs, back)		
Body part	**Exercise**	**Sets**	**Reps**
Warm up with a 5-minute cardiovascular activity and some mobility movements			
Legs	Squat	4	8, 6, 3–4, 3–4
	Dead lift	4	8, 6, 3–4, 3–4
Upper back	Bent-over row	4	8, 6, 3–4, 3–4
	Lat pull-down	4	8, 6, 3–4, 3–4
Abdominals	Roll-out with ball	2	12–15
	Hanging leg raise	2	12–15

Table 21.2	Strength workout 2 (chest, shoulders, arms)		
Body part	**Exercise**	**Sets**	**Reps**
Warm up with a 5-minute cardiovascular activity and some mobility movements			
Chest	Bench press	4	8, 6, 3–4, 3–4
	Incline dumbbell press	4	8, 6, 3–4, 3–4
Shoulders	Dumbbell press	4	8, 6, 3–4, 3–4
	Upright row	4	8, 6, 3–4, 3–4
Abdominals	Oblique crunch	2	12–15
	Exercise ball jackknife/pike	2	12–15

BODY WEIGHT WORKOUTS

22

You don't always need weights or equipment to build strength. Your own body is the most versatile piece of resistance training equipment you'll ever own! Squats, push-ups, lunges, crunches – there are plenty of exercises that utilise your own body weight and gravity, and these can form part of your regular strength training programme. Make use of them on days when you can't get to the gym, or don't have access to equipment; or incorporate them into your programme when you simply want a change from your usual weights routine.

Here are three body-weight workouts that work all the major muscle groups. They are based on the principle of peripheral heart action training, which conditions the muscles and increases cardiovascular fitness at the same time. Alternating upper and lower body exercises with minimal rest periods between each exercise places greater demands on the cardiovascular system than conventional resistance training workouts. It also burns more calories per minute so is particularly beneficial if you want to reduce (or prevent gaining) body fat. It means you get the dual benefits of increased strength and increased cardiovascular fitness.

WARM UP AND COOL DOWN

Always warm up with 5–10 minutes cardiovascular exercise before your workout to reduce your risk of injury. After completing your workout, spend 5 minutes stretching.

HOW MANY REPS?

Do the prescribed number of reps for each exercise. Perform the exercises consecutively with 30 seconds' rest in between.

HOW MANY CIRCUITS?

Do 1–2 circuits, taking 60–90 seconds' rest between circuits. You may increase the number of circuits depending on the time you have available.

Table 22.1	Body weight workout 1
Exercise	**Reps**
Body weight squat on BOSU	12–15
V-sits	12–15
Bench dip	12–15
Lunge twist	12–15
Push-ups	12–15
BOSU plank	Hold for 30–60 seconds
Mountain climbers	12–15
Side bridge/plank	Hold for 30–60 seconds

Table 22.3	Body weight workout 3
Exercise	**Reps**
Split squat jumps	12–15
Medicine ball twist	12–15
Single leg dead lift	12–15
Push-up (feet elevated)	12–15
Exercise ball jackknife	12–15
Bench dip	12–15
Single leg split squat (rear foot on BOSU/step)	12–15
Plank (single arm)	Hold for 60–120 seconds

Table 22.2	Body weight workout 2
Exercise	**Reps**
Squat jumps	12–15
Pull-up	8–10
Roll-out with ball	12–15
Front lunge	12–15
Push-up (close grip)	12–15
Plank (feet elevated)	Hold for 60 seconds
Side lunge	12–15
Side bridge/plank	Hold for 60 seconds

POWER WORKOUTS

23

Power or plyometric workouts are designed to increase muscular power and explosiveness. They can help improve your performance in many sports, including track and field athletics, football, rugby, basketball, martial arts and racket sports. Plyometric exercises are usually done with body weight or very light loads such as plyo push-ups, box jumps and jump squats. The idea is to train for maximum force production in the smallest period of time, so reps are kept low and the intensity and effort is high.

Plyometric training is based on the principle that a concentric muscular action is much stronger immediately following an eccentric action of the same muscle. The muscles are able to store the tension from the stretch for a short period of time – causing the muscle to react like a rubber band. The greatest force can be achieved when the stretch is performed as fast as possible.

There are many benefits of plyometric training, including enhanced performance, explosive power, eccentric strength, coordination and reduced injury risk in sport. It can increase your vertical jump height, boost your running speed and help you throw further. In swimming, it can help you push off the blocks more explosively as well as improve your turns.

Plyometric training not only improves sports performance, it can also help build muscle. That's because it engages the FT muscle fibres, thus increasing their strength and efficiency.

Due to the high impact nature of most plyometric exercises, only well-conditioned lifters and athletes should use this type of training as it carries a higher risk of injury. You need good muscle strength and joint stability as well as good technique to perform the exercises effectively.

You can add plyometric exercises to the beginning or end of your weights workout or substitute your usual weights workout with a plyometric workout. Start with just 1 or 2 exercises then progress gradually, adding more exercises or sets to your workout as you become accustomed to the movements. Do not attempt to do plyometric training in every workout as it can cause a high degree of stress and inflammation to your muscles. You will almost certainly experience delayed onset muscle soreness (DOMS) after a power workout but this should lessen over time. Do just one power workout a week initially, increasing gradually to 2 sessions a week. Here are three total-body workouts based on different training methods.

WARM UP

Warm up with 5–10 minutes of cardiovascular activity and some drills that replicate the movements you are about to perform.

BODY WEIGHT POWER WORKOUT

This workout is based on body weight exercises that help develop total-body power. Do the prescribed number of repetitions, taking 30 seconds' rest between exercises. After completing the first circuit, take 2–3 minutes' rest. Repeat the circuit once, building up to 3 circuits as you get accustomed to power training.

Table 23.1	Body weight power workout
Exercise	**Reps**
Burpees	10–15
Squat jump	10–15
Split squats	10–15
Alternating plyo push-ups	10–15
Mountain climbers	10–15

JUMPING WORKOUT

This workout develops lower body power and will help increase jumping and sprinting abilities. Perform bunny hops over a set distance and complete the prescribed number of repetitions for the box jumps, taking 2–3 minutes' rest between each exercise. Rest for 2–3 minutes after the first circuit then repeat once or twice, depending on your level of conditioning. Start with one circuit then gradually build to 2 or 3 circuits as you get accustomed to power training.

Table 23.2	Jumping workout
Exercise	**Reps**
Bunny hops	30–50
Box jump (depth jump)	10–15
Vertical depth jump	10–15

MEDICINE BALL POWER WORKOUT

This workout with a medicine ball develops total-body power. Select a ball between 2 and 5 kg in weight, depending on your strength. As you get stronger, increase the weight of medicine ball used. Do the prescribed number of repetitions, taking 30 seconds' rest between exercises. After completing the first circuit, take 2–3 minutes rest. Repeat once, building up to 3 circuits as you get accustomed to power training.

Table 23.3	Medicine ball power workout
Exercise	**Reps**
Chest throw	10–20
Seated overhead throw	10–20
Standing throw to floor	10–20

POWER WORKOUTS

TRAINING FOR SPORTS PROGRAMMES

24

While fitness athletes and bodybuilders train primarily to change the appearance of their physiques, other athletes can tailor a strength training programme to improve various aspects of their sports performance.

Resistance training can help to:

- improve sports performance
- improve strength, power, muscle size or muscular endurance
- reduce injury risk.

General guidelines for strength training for sport

1. Use different programmes for each season, focusing on developing only one of these goals (e.g. strength). Attempting to improve in two or more areas (e.g. strength and muscular endurance) simultaneously will produce only mediocre improvements.

2. During the off-season, focus on developing your strength and hypertrophy.

3. Pre-season training should focus on one particular fitness aspect (e.g. power, muscular endurance or strength) that is relevant to the sport. Use one of the programmes detailed in the first part of this chapter.

4. During the season, concentrate on maintaining your fitness and staying injury-free. The frequency and duration of your strength training workouts should be reduced and the exercises should be more sport-specific.

5. Include mostly compound exercises in your programme. They will improve your balance and coordination while increasing strength. Keep isolation exercises to a minimum and schedule these at the end of your workout.

6. Keep rest periods fairly short (between 60 and 90 seconds) to mimic the demands of your sport.

7. Choose a weight with which the set becomes difficult by the last 1 or 2 repetitions.

8. Maintain strict form for each repetition, using the complete ROM.

9. Emphasise quality rather than quantity.

When designing a sports strength training programme, however, it has to be specific to the requirements of your sport. You need to consider the following:

- the movement patterns of your sport, and which muscles are used
- the relative importance of strength, power, hypertrophy and muscular endurance in your sport
- which muscles or joints are most prone to injury and therefore need strengthening
- the priorities of your sport's season – i.e. off-season, pre-season, in-season and post-season
- your fitness level and training experience.

THE ATHLETE'S (SPRINTER'S) WORKOUT

GOAL

This workout includes exercises for each muscle group, with a particular emphasis on compound exercises, to cause maximum muscle stimulation. There is equal emphasis on lower- and upper-body exercises to build balanced muscle development. Moderate to heavy weights should be used, and the prescribed sets and reps are designed to develop muscle strength and hypertrophy.

IN-SEASON GUIDELINES

As the competitive season approaches, reduce the number of resistance training sessions to twice a week and increase the time spent on sport-specific training.

Increase the number of repetitions to 12–15 to emphasise muscle endurance.

Include plyometrics and jump exercises after a good warm-up, then follow with strength exercises. Do approximately 10 reps per set with a 3–5 minute rest between sets.

Table 24.1	Priorities for a sport-specific strength training programme		
Season	**Sports-specific training**	**Strength training**	**Strength-training goal**
Off-season	Low	High	Hypertrophy and strength
Pre-season	Medium	Medium	Strength/power/muscular endurance – depending on the sport
In-season	High	Low	Maintain strength/power/muscular endurance

Table 24.2	Athlete's (sprinter's) workout		
Muscle group	**Exercise**	**Sets**	**Reps**
Workout 1 (lower body)			
Quadriceps/gluteals	Squat	2–3	8–12
	Dead lift	2–3	8–12
Quadriceps/gluteals/hamstrings	Lunge (front or reverse)	2	8–12
Hamstrings	Straight leg dead lift	2	8–12
Calves	Standing calf raise	3	8–12
Abdominals	Crunch	2	15–20
	Hanging leg raise	2	15–20
Workout 2 (upper body)			
Chest	Bench press (flat or incline)	2–3	8–12
Back	Bent-over row	2–3	8–12
Shoulders	Shoulder press (barbell/dumbbell)	2–3	8–12
Biceps	Barbell curl	2	8–12
Triceps	Lying triceps extension	2	8–12
Trapezius	Dumbbell shrug	2	8–12
Lower back	Back extension	2	12–15
Abdominals	Cable rotation	2	15–20
	Plank	2	Hold for 60 seconds

THE FOOTBALLER'S WORKOUT

GOAL

This workout aims to develop overall strength and hypertrophy. It therefore includes exercises for each muscle group to promote balanced development, as all muscles are important in football. Rather more emphasis (in the form of more sets) is placed on exercises for the lower body, in particular exercises for the hamstrings, than the upper body.

IN-SEASON GUIDELINES

As the competitive season approaches, reduce resistance training sessions to twice a week and increase the time spent on sport-specific training.

Reduce the number of sets per body part and increase the number of repetitions to 12–15 to emphasise muscle endurance. Include plyometrics and jump exercises after a good warm-up, then follow with strength exercises. Do approximately 10 reps per set with a 3–5 minute rest between sets.

Table 24.3	Footballer's workout		
Muscle group	**Exercise**	**Sets**	**Reps**
Workout 1 (lower body)			
Quadriceps/gluteals	Leg press	3	8–12
Quadriceps	Leg extension	3	8–12
Hamstrings	Seated leg curl	3	8–12
Calves	Standing calf raise	3	8–12
Lower back	Back extension	2	12–15
Abdominals	Medicine ball twist	2	15–20
	Hanging leg raise	2	15–20
Workout 2 (upper body)			
Chest	Bench press (flat or incline)	3	8–12
Back	Lat pull-down	3	8–12
Shoulders	Dumbbell shoulder press	3	8–12
Triceps	Lying triceps extension	3	8–12
Biceps	Barbell curl	3	8–12
Abdominals	Oblique crunch	2	12–15
	Exercise ball jackknife	2	12–15

THE SWIMMER'S WORKOUT

GOAL

This workout aims to develop muscular and cardiovascular endurance as well as some strength. It emphasises exercises for the upper body, since arm action is the most important action for generating speed in swimming, and exercises for the midsection as these muscles are important for maintaining the straight-body water position. It also includes a plyometric exercise for legs to help improve the explosive power needed for push-offs.

For general conditioning, do 12–15 reps per set with 30–60 seconds' rest in between sets. Sprinters may wish to do fewer reps and use heavier weights to build strength; long-distance swimmers may wish to do a higher number of reps, around 15–20.

IN-SEASON GUIDELINES

As the competitive season approaches, reduce resistance training sessions to twice a week and increase the time spent on sport-specific training – movements that duplicate the movement patterns of each stroke – and in the pool. You can adapt many resistance training exercises to mimic the actions in a particular stroke more closely.

Include more plyometric exercises after a good warm-up, then follow with strength exercises. Do approximately 10 reps per set with a 3–5 minute rest between sets.

Table 24.4	Swimmer's workout		
Muscle group	**Exercise**	**Sets**	**Reps**
Back	Pull-down	3	12–15
	Dumbbell pull-over	3	12–15
Shoulders	Bent-over lateral raise	3	12–15
	Dumbbell lateral raise	3	12–15
Biceps	Barbell curl	2	12–15
Triceps	Triceps press-down	2	12–15
Lower back	Superman	2	12–15
Lower body	Squat jumps (with or without dumbbells)	2	10–12
Abdominals	Roll-out with ball	2	15–20
	Medicine ball twist	2	15–20
	Exercise ball pull-in	2	15–20

THE RUGBY PLAYER'S WORKOUT

GOAL

Rugby players require considerable strength, power and speed as well as endurance. This workout focuses on strength, power and hypertrophy and includes basic compound exercises for both upper and lower body to promote balanced development.

IN-SEASON GUIDELINES

As the competitive season approaches, reduce the number of resistance training sessions to twice a week and increase the time spent on sport-specific training.

Reduce the number of sets per body part and increase the number of repetitions to 12–15 to emphasise muscle endurance.

Include plyometric and jump exercises after a good warm-up, then follow with strength

Table 24.5	Rugby player's workout		
Muscle group	**Exercise**	**Sets**	**Reps**
Workout 1 (lower body, back)			
Lower body	Squat	3	6–10
	Dead lift	3	6–10
Quadriceps	Leg extension	2	6–10
Hamstrings	Lying leg curl	2	6–10
Calves	Standing calf raise	3	6–10
	Seated calf raise	3	6–10
Back	Bent-over barbell row	3	6–10
	Pull-up/chin-up	3	6–10
Lower back	Back extension on machine	2	12–15
Abdominals	Hanging leg raise	2	12–15
	Reverse crunch	2	12–15
Workout 2 (chest, shoulders, arms)			
Chest	Bench press	3	6–10
	Incline dumbbell press	3	6–10
Shoulders	Dumbbell shoulder press	3	6–10
	Upright row	3	6–10
Triceps	Lying triceps extension	3	6–10
Biceps	Barbell curl	3	6–10
Abdominals	Oblique crunch	2	12–15
	Exercise ball pull-in	2	12–15

TRAINING FOR SPORTS PROGRAMMES

exercises. Do approximately 10 reps per set with a 3–5 minute rest between sets.

THE RUNNER'S WORKOUT

GOAL

The aim of this workout is to improve overall conditioning. It develops your muscular and cardiovascular endurance and provides a balanced workout to help avoid the overuse injuries that are common in running.

IN-SEASON GUIDELINES

As the competitive season approaches, reduce the number of resistance training sessions to twice a week and increase running training. Increase the reps and reduce the weights.

Table 24.6	Runner's workout		
Muscle group	**Exercise**	**Sets**	**Reps**
Legs	Split squat	2	12–15
	Step-ups	2	12–15
Calves	Calf raise	2	12–15
Chest	Dumbbell flye	2	12–15
Shoulders	Lateral raise	2	12–15
Back	Lat pull-down	2	12–15
Biceps	Dumbbell curl	2	12–15
Triceps	Triceps press-down	2	12–15
Lower back	Back extension	2	12–15
Abdominals	Reverse crunch	2	15–20
	Plank	2	Hold for 60–90 seconds

THE CYCLIST'S WORKOUT

GOAL

The aim of this workout is to increase your muscular and cardiovascular endurance. It includes exercises for the upper and lower body to provide balanced development. You should also spend at least 15 minutes stretching 3 times a week, focusing on the lower back.

IN-SEASON GUIDELINES

As the competitive season approaches, reduce the number of resistance training sessions to twice a week and increase time spent in the saddle.

Increase the number of reps and reduce the weights.

Table 24.7	Cyclist's workout		
Muscle group	**Exercise**	**Sets**	**Reps**
Shoulders	Overhead press machine	3	12–15
Back	Lat pull-down	3	12–15
Chest	Vertical bench press machine	3	12–15
Legs	Front or reverse lunge	3	12–15
Hamstrings	Seated leg curl	3	12–15
Lower back	Back extension	2	12–15
Calves	Seated calf raise	3	12–15
Abdominals	Exercise ball crunch	2	15–20
	Hip thrust	2	15–20

THE MARTIAL ARTIST'S WORKOUT

GOAL

Martial artists require strength, explosive power and speed as well as endurance. This workout includes exercises for each muscle group. Perform your exercises in an explosive manner, focusing on lifting the weight (i.e. the concentric part of the movement) as fast as possible.

IN-SEASON GUIDELINES

As the competitive season approaches, reduce the number of resistance training sessions to twice a week and increase the time spent on sport-specific training.

Reduce the number of sets per body part and increase the number of repetitions to 12–15 to emphasise muscle endurance.

Include plyometric and jump exercises after a good warm-up, then follow with strength exercises. Do approximately 10 reps per set with a 3–5 minute rest between sets.

Table 24.8	Martial artist's workout		
Muscle group	**Exercise**	**Sets**	**Reps**
Workout 1 (lower body, back)			
Lower body	Squat jump	3	8–10
Quadriceps	Leg extension	2	8–10
Hamstrings	Seated leg curl	2	8–10
Calves	Standing calf raise	3	8–10
Back	Pull-up/chin-up	3	8–10
	One arm dumbbell row	2	8–10
Lower back	Back extension	2	8–10
Abdominals	Exercise ball crunch	2	12–15
	Side bridge	2	Hold for 5 seconds, repeat 5 times
Workout 2 (chest, shoulders, arms)			
Chest	Bench press	3	8–10
	Incline dumbbell press	3	8–10
Shoulders	Dumbbell shoulder press	3	8–10
	Dumbbell lateral raise	3	8–10
Triceps	Lying triceps extension	3	8–10
Biceps	Barbell curl	3	8–10
Abdominals	Oblique crunch	2	12–15
	Exercise ball jackknife	2	12–15

THE TENNIS PLAYER'S WORKOUT

GOAL

This workout will increase your muscular endurance and develop some strength. It includes exercises for both the upper and lower body, but focuses on exercises for the shoulders and back.

IN-SEASON GUIDELINES

As the competitive season approaches, increase the reps to 15–20 and reduce the weights. Spend more time doing sport-specific training.

Table 24.9	Tennis player's workout		
Muscle group	**Exercise**	**Sets**	**Reps**
Shoulders	Overhead press machine	3	10–12
Back	Dumbbell pull-over	3	10–12
Shoulders	Cable lateral raise	3	10–12
Back	Seated cable row	3	10–12
Chest	Pec-deck flye	3	10–12
Legs	Front or reverse lunge	3	10–12
Lower back	Back extension	2	12–15
Calves	Standing calf raise	3	12–15
Abdominals	Exercise ball crunch	2	12–15
	Medicine ball twist	2	12–15

THE CARDIOVASCULAR PROGRAMME

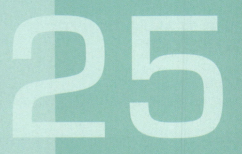

It is not possible to build muscle and lose fat simultaneously. But, over time, you can increase your muscle mass and cut fat gradually. The key is to incorporate cardiovascular exercise training in your resistance training programme and pay careful attention to your diet.

Cardiovascular exercise not only burns calories while you are working out but also increases your body's ability to burn fat the rest of the time. Contrary to popular belief, cardiovascular exercise is not counterproductive to a resistance training programme. It will not burn hard-earned muscle nor prevent gains in muscle size. In fact, cardiovascular training is essential for any fitness or sports training programme, not just for fat burning but also for its performance- and immunity-boosting effects.

THE BENEFITS OF CARDIO-VASCULAR TRAINING

Cardiovascular training:

- reduces body fat and maintains a low body fat percentage
- increases the body's fat-burning capacity during exercise and rest
- improves body composition
- increases the metabolic rate
- reduces stress and anxiety
- improves confidence, self-esteem and mood
- reduces blood pressure, blood cholesterol and the risk of heart disease
- boosts the immune system.

THE SCIENCE BIT ...

Regular cardiovascular training increases the body's ability to break down fat by increasing the production of hormone-dependent lipase. This enzyme breaks down fat into its component fatty acids, which are then transported in the bloodstream to the muscles, where they can be broken down to release energy. The better conditioned you are, the higher your levels of fat-burning enzymes and so the more fat you can burn at rest or during exercise. Just as you can train your muscles to become stronger and bigger, so you can train your aerobic system to burn fat more efficiently.

The benefits of cardiovascular training don't end with your workout. Following exercise, your metabolic rate remains elevated for some time as your body replenishes its energy systems. This 'excess post-exercise oxygen consumption' (EPOC) is fuelled almost entirely by fat. Following low-intensity training, the EPOC is very small but following high-intensity training it may be quite large.

DESIGNING YOUR CARDIO-VASCULAR PROGRAMME

WHICH ACTIVITY?

Cardiovascular exercise includes any kind of activity that uses the large muscle groups of the body and can be kept up for 20–40 minutes, with your heart rate in your target training range (60–85 per cent of maximum heart rate):

- running/treadmill
- fitness/power walking
- stepping machine/stair climber
- cycling/stationary bicycle
- swimming
- aerobic classes/aqua aerobics/step aerobics
- climbing machine
- elliptical training machine
- rowing machine.

The choice depends on your personal preference, and the equipment and time available to you. It's important to plan your workouts around activities that you enjoy, and also to vary the exercise mode as far as possible. The more enthusiastic you are about an activity, the more likely you are to work hard and keep it up. In fact, frequently changing the mode of cardio may produce better results than simply increasing the duration of time you spend doing it as your body becomes more efficient in performing a movement over time, using less energy.

HOW MUCH AND HOW OFTEN?

ACSM recommends 150 minutes per week to improve cardiovascular health or 200–300 minutes to lose weight (Garber et al, 2011). This can be met through 30-60 minutes of moderate-intensity exercise (5 days per week) or 20-60 minutes of vigorous-intensity exercise (3 days per week). Increase the intensity and duration of your sessions gradually, aiming for 60 minutes 5 times a week.

HOW INTENSE?

The harder you train, the more calories you burn. As a guide, you should be working within your target heart rate zone (THR), which is between 60 and 85 per cent of your maximum heart rate (MHR). Your MHR is the highest heart rate value you can achieve in an all-out effort to the point of exhaustion. It remains constant from day to day and decreases only slightly from year to year – by about one beat per year beginning at 10–15 years of age.

To estimate your MHR, subtract your age from 220. For example, if you were 30, your MHR would be estimated at 190 beats per minute (bpm):

MHR = 220 – 30 = 190 beats per minute
THR zone = (60% x 190) – (85% x 190)
= 114–162 beats per minute

So, in training, the 30-year-old in the example above should aim to keep his or her heart rate above 114 bpm but below 162 bpm (your lower and upper figures will, of course, depend on using your own age in the above calculation). If you train above your THR zone you begin to work anaerobically and your body can't keep up with the demand for oxygen. You won't be able to sustain this workout intensity very long and will soon reach fatigue. Work within your THR zone to get maximum cardiovascular benefit from your workout.

Whether you choose a high- or low-intensity cardiovascular programme depends on your goals, fitness level and time available. Both types will develop cardiovascular fitness and burn fat but high-intensity exercise (over 70 per cent of your MHR) is more efficient. If time is at a premium, shorter periods of high-intensity exercise will give you the same results in terms of fat loss as longer periods of low-intensity cardio. Training at the lower end of the THR zone is better for beginners and is certainly more attractive for many casual exercisers.

HOW SHOULD I MONITOR MY HEART RATE?

The best way to monitor your heart rate during your workout is to use a heart rate monitor or take your pulse manually. You can also use the rate of perceived exertion (RPE) scale. This is a subjective rating of how hard you feel you are exercising. The most popular version of this is the Borg scale, a modified version of which is shown in Table 25.1. This 10-point scale ranges from 1 (nothing at all) to 10 (maximum effort). Used correctly, it is a very accurate system for monitoring exercise intensity.

STEADY PACE OR INTERVALS?

Steady pace training – keeping your heart rate fairly constant throughout your workout – builds endurance and a good base level of fitness. High-intensity interval training (HIIT) – exercising for short periods at a high intensity, interspersed

The fat-burning zone myth

It's a long-held belief that low-intensity cardiovascular exercise – equivalent to brisk walking or jogging – is the best way to burn fat. It is based on the observation that low-intensity exercise burns a greater percentage of calories from fat than from carbohydrate (Phillips et al, 1996). In fact, the body burns more fat (as opposed to percentage fat in the fuel mixture) during higher-intensity cardiovascular exercise because the rate of calorie expenditure is higher. It is not the proportion of each fuel metabolised but the total calorie expenditure that is most important. For example, walking (low-intensity cardio) for 60 minutes will burn about 270 kcal, of which approximately 60 per cent (160 kcal) comes from fat, while jogging (high-intensity cardio) for 60 minutes will burn about 680 kcal, of which approximately 40 per cent (270 kcal) comes from fat. Thus, the higher-intensity exercise results in a greater fat loss over the same workout time.

with lower-intensity recovery periods – builds cardiovascular strength and stamina. The heart and lungs are worked harder during this type of training so they will become stronger and, as a result, you become fitter. It is a more effective way of burning fat than steady pace training because it produces a greater 'after burn' or EPOC, and speeds up your metabolic rate for up to 18 hours after your workout (Smith & McNaughton, 1993). A study carried out at McMaster University found that HIIT performed 3 times a week produced similar fitness gains to doing steady state training

5 times a week (Little et al, 2010). A review of 37 different studies on interval training and aerobic fitness concluded that HIIT is an effective method of increasing cardiovascular fitness as measured by VO_2max (Bacon et al, 2013).

Both types of training can easily be applied to any mode of cardiovascular exercise – running, cycling, stationary bike, stepping machine, elliptical trainer or any other cardio machine. During the interval phases, you increase either your speed or the resistance of the machine (e.g. the incline of a treadmill or the resistance – 'level' – setting on a stationary bike) in order to reach the required RPE level of 8–9, or 80–90 per cent MHR. This is maintained for 15 seconds to 3 minutes, depending on the intensity, followed by a recovery period at an RPE of 4 (somewhat hard) or 60 per cent MHR for 30 seconds to 3 minutes.

TOO MUCH CARDIO?

More isn't always better, as excessive cardiovascular exercise can result in muscle breakdown

High-intensity cardiovascular exercise – this is generally accepted as an intensity corresponding to more than 75 per cent MHR.

Low-intensity cardiovascular exercise – this is generally accepted as an intensity corresponding to less than 75 per cent MHR.

and a loss of muscle size and strength. During cardiovascular training, protein can be used for energy, although the misconception that it significantly depletes muscle mass relates more directly to poor diet. An inadequate calorie intake together with high-volume cardiovascular training can result in significant muscle breakdown.

This is induced by the release of the catabolic hormone cortisol (released during all types of high-intensity activity), which outstrips the production of anabolic hormones such as testosterone. Under

Table 25.1	Rating of perceived exertion (RPE)		
At rest		1	Non-exercise HR*
Light activity – sitting working		2	Non-exercise HR
Light activity – walking at leisurely pace		3	Non-exercise HR
Moderate activity – purposeful walking		4	Non-exercise HR
Moderate activity – brisk walking		5	Non-exercise HR
Somewhat hard activity – jogging		6	60% MHR**
Hard activity – running, breathing harder		7	65–75% MHR
Very hard activity – running, conversation just possible		8	80% MHR
Very very hard activity – fast running, conversation difficult		9	85% MHR
Maximum effort – unable to speak		10	MHR

* heart rate
** maximum heart rate

these conditions there is a net catabolism, or breakdown, of muscle tissue. One study measured a decrease in the size of FT fibres following a 3-month period of aerobic training on a treadmill (Kraemer *et al*, 1995). This may help explain the low muscle mass of many endurance runners.

Dieters who go overboard with cardiovascular training don't realise that a large proportion of their weight loss may be due to muscle loss. When the body doesn't get enough calories it draws upon its reserves, mainly in the form of fat but also from protein, which is found in muscle. You can end up cannibalising your own muscle tissue to help your body meet its energy needs. That's the last thing a strength trainer wants.

For this reason, cardio should be done in moderation, as per the guidelines above. Moderate amounts of cardio will help you lose fat, and give you numerous health benefits.

WHAT IS THE BEST TIME FOR CARDIOVASCULAR TRAINING?

This depends on your individual lifestyle. Choose a time of day that fits in well with your daily schedule; that way you will be less likely to miss a workout. Research suggests that it may be better to perform your cardio and strength training as separate sessions to minimise catabolism (the breakdown of lean mass), but if you prefer to do both in one session, complete your resistance training workout first when glycogen stores are high. Performing cardio prior to your strength training workout may be counterproductive, resulting in reduced strength and early fatigue due to muscle glycogen depletion.

RESISTANCE TRAINING BURNS FAT TOO

It's not only cardio that burns body fat – resistance training will also help you get lean (Osterberg & Melby, 2000). Researchers at Colorado State University measured the RMR of volunteers following an hour's strenuous resistance training and discovered that their RMRs remained significantly elevated for 3 hours after the workout. Even after 16 hours the RMR remained a little higher than normal, as did the rate of fat oxidation. Since RMR makes up the major proportion (60–70 per cent) of total daily energy expenditure, any increase in RMR would have a big impact on your daily calorie output. Therefore, regular strenuous resistance training workouts are an effective strategy for upping calorie burning and losing fat.

STEADY-PACE CARDIO-VASCULAR WORKOUT 1

Workout time: 30–50 min (including warm-up and cool-down)
THR zone: 60–75 per cent MHR
RPE: 6–7 (moderate)

This workout is suitable for beginners. Start with a 5-minute warm-up, then gradually build up your pace or machine resistance until you reach your training zone (60–75 per cent MHR) or an RPE of 6–7 (moderate). Maintain your intensity in this zone for 20–40 minutes, depending on your fitness and time available. Gradually reduce your pace or resistance for a 5-minute cool-down before stretching out.

STEADY-PACE CARDIO-VASCULAR WORKOUT 2

Workout time: 30–50 min (including warm-up and cool-down)

THR zone: 75–85 per cent MHR

RPE: 8 (hard–very hard)

This workout is suitable for well-conditioned trainers only. Start with a 5-minute warm-up, then gradually build up your pace or machine resistance until you reach your training zone (75–85 per cent MHR) or an RPE of 8 (hard or very hard). Maintain your intensity in this zone for 20–40 minutes. Gradually reduce your pace or resistance for a 5-minute cool-down before stretching out.

INTERVAL TRAINING CARDIO-VASCULAR WORKOUT

Workout time: 30–50 min (including warm-up and cool-down)

THR zone: 80–90 per cent MHR for high-intensity intervals; 60–65 per cent MHR for low-intensity intervals

RPE: 8–9 (very hard) for high-intensity intervals; 6 (somewhat hard) for low-intensity intervals

This workout is suitable for very well-conditioned trainers only but is a very efficient way to burn fat. Start with a 5-minute warm-up, then perform 9 sets of 2-minute intervals. Adjust your pace or machine resistance to reach your training zone (80–90 per cent MHR) or an RPE of 8–9 for 1 minute, followed by 1 or 2 minutes at 60–65 per cent MHR or an RPE of 6. Gradually reduce your pace or resistance for a 5-minute cool-down before stretching out.

SUMMARY OF KEY POINTS

- It is important to include cardio training in a strength training programme to improve body composition, increase the RMR and improve cardiovascular fitness.
- Cardiovascular fitness is developed by performing 3–5 cardiovascular training sessions lasting 20–40 minutes per week.
- High-intensity cardiovascular exercise is more effective than low-intensity cardiovascular exercise for burning body fat and developing cardiovascular fitness.
- Interval training is more effective than steady pace training for developing cardiovascular fitness.
- Excessive cardiovascular exercise with an inadequate calorie intake can result in muscle breakdown and loss of muscle mass.

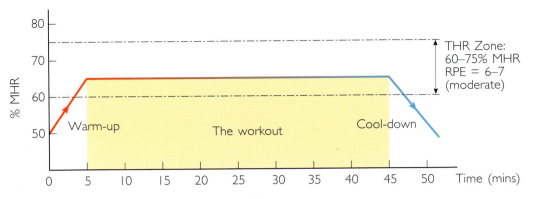

Figure 25.1 Steady-pace cardiovascular workout 1

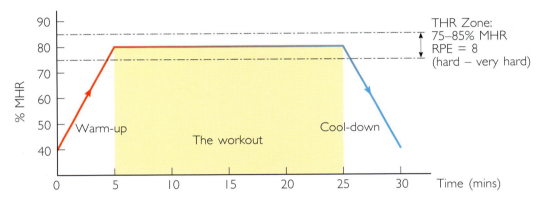

Figure 25.2 Steady-pace cardiovascular workout 2

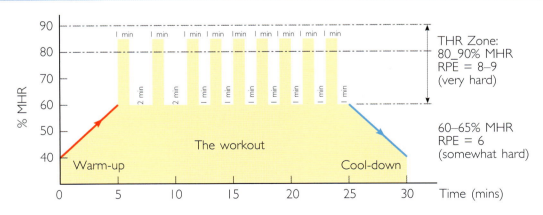

Figure 25.3 Interval training cardiovascular workout

TRAINING FOR SPECIFIC RESULTS

26

You cannot change your basic shape, which is determined by your genes, but with resistance training you can refine your dimensions and develop your physique to its best potential.

This chapter shows you how to re-sculpt your body through specific training programmes. Whether you are naturally thin or stocky, you can improve your shape by following the training guidelines for your body type and for specific body parts.

BODY TYPES

The Sheldon system classifies body types into three basic categories:

1. ectomorph
2. mesomorph
3. endomorph.

Most people are a mixture of these three types but tend to resemble one type more strongly. For example, you may share most of the characteristics

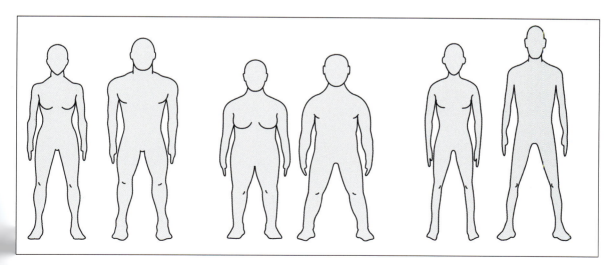

Figure 26.1 Sheldon body types. Mesomorph (left); endomorph (centre); ectomorph right).

253

of a mesomorph (wide shoulders and narrow hips) but have slight endomorphic tendencies as well (gain fat readily).

The ectomorph is lean and thin with little muscle bulk and low body-fat levels. This person has narrow shoulders and hips, and a fast metabolism, which makes it difficult to gain muscle or fat. At the other end of the spectrum, the endomorph has a naturally stocky, rounded build with wide shoulders and wide hips. This person has an even distribution of fat and gains both muscle and fat easily, making training gains less visible. The mesomorph has a naturally athletic build with wide shoulders and narrow hips. This person gains muscle readily and finds it easy to shed fat, so tends to make the best bodybuilder.

HOW SHOULD AN ECTOMORPH TRAIN?

If you are an ectomorph, your muscle gains will be slower than those of the other body types. Realistically, you cannot expect to gain much more than 0.5 kg/month, although you may gain muscle faster during the first 3–6 months. However, don't be discouraged if your gains come slowly – the beginner's programme (p. 210) will help you develop a good foundation of strength. Progress to the intermediate's programme (p. 217) to increase muscle size and strength, concentrating on basic compound movements such as squats, bench presses and dead lifts. These exercises will stimulate larger amounts of muscle mass and a greater number of muscle fibres. Keep isolation exercises to a minimum, and limit your cardiovascular training to two sessions/week, opting for low-intensity rather than high-intensity training (seepp. 249). Also follow the weight-gain eating tips (p. 77).

HOW SHOULD AN ENDOMORPH TRAIN?

Endomorphs are naturally strong and generally have little trouble gaining muscle and strength. However, your gains may be hidden under a layer of fat, so the main focus of your training programme should be fat-burning cardiovascular activity. Aim to perform a cardiovascular workout 3–6 days/week, including at least two high-intensity interval workouts (see p. 251) in addition to your strength training. High-intensity cardiovascular training burns more fat than low-intensity training both during your workout and afterwards. If you do your cardio workout first thing in the morning, your muscles will also burn more calories from fat. Another way to encourage fat being used for fuel is to avoid eating carbohydrate shortly before your workouts in order to keep insulin levels in your bloodstream low. Following your workouts, wait 1 hour before eating in order to encourage more fat to be broken down to replenish short-term energy stores. Follow the beginner's programme (see p. 210) to increase muscular endurance and muscle tone – this will give you a good base of strength and a lower body-fat percentage. As your fitness improves, increase the number of circuits, sets and repetitions – this will burn more calories.

HOW SHOULD A MESOMORPH TRAIN?

As a mesomorph, you tend to get good gains from just about anything you do in the gym. However, that's not to say that you can train mindlessly. A well-designed programme will keep you focused and optimise your gains. The key is to use a periodised programme, breaking your training into shorter cycles to achieve year-round gains in strength and size (see p. 30). This will help you avoid overtraining. You should vary your routines frequently, using advanced training techniques such as supersets and descending sets once you have sufficient experience. Change the order of your exercises, the number of sets and repetitions, and the rest intervals used to provide plenty of variety and increase your motivation. Your workout can include a mixture of compound and isolation exercises, and should include cardio training 3 times per week to keep your body-fat levels low and improve your cardiovascular fitness. Follow the beginner's and intermediate's programmes (see pp. 210 and 217), progressing to the advanced workouts (see p. 223) once you have at least 1 year's training experience.

WHAT IS MY OPTIMAL BODY-FAT PERCENTAGE?

It is impossible to set an optimal body-fat percentage that applies to everyone. The body-fat level that your body comfortably reaches without strict dieting is dependent on your genetic make-up as well as your diet and activity. Your natural body type dictates to some extent how much fat you carry and how readily you store it. For example, if you are an ectomorph or meso-morph, you are naturally lean and will be able to achieve a lower body-fat percentage than an endo-morph who stores fat easily. But, whatever your natural body type, you can still achieve a lower body-fat level and more defined physique through consistent hard training and healthy eating. The important point is to decide on a level that is realistic for your build and shape.

HOW LOW CAN I GO?

Healthy ranges for the general population are 18–25 per cent for women and 13–18 per cent for men. But if you are a strength trainer or bodybuilder, you may desire lower levels. Between 10 per cent and 20 per cent for women, and between 6 per cent and 15 per cent for men are common among well-trained athletes – levels that are generally associated with peak performance – but these percentages should be regarded with some caution. If you try to attain a low body-fat percentage that is unnatural for your genetic make-up, you may encounter problems.

For women, a body-fat percentage that is under their individual threshold for menstrua-tion (14–20 per cent) can be risky. Below this, a deficiency of oestrogen and progesterone similar to those levels experienced during and after the menopause can result in amenorrhoea (cessation of menstruation). This can lead to infertility, loss of bone density, stress fractures and premature osteoporosis. Most experts therefore recommend a lower limit of 14 per cent body fat for women.

If a man's body-fat percentage dips too low, there are health risks too. Studies have shown that when men reach a body-fat level of 4–6 per cent, their bodies start to feed on muscle tissue as a source of energy and to allow them to maintain their fat stores at a minimal level (Friedl *et al*, 1994). It is definitely unwise, if not impossible, to reduce your body fat below this level. Other studies have found that testosterone levels plummet below 5 per cent body fat, causing reduced sexual drive and fertility (Strauss *et al*, 1993).

LEG CLINIC

SYMMETRY PROBLEM: THIN LEGS AND DIFFICULTY GAINING SIZE

Skinny legs produce an overall weak appearance. The symmetry problem is exacerbated if you have a well-developed upper body – a particularly common fault in men who put more emphasis on training their chest, shoulders and arms but neglect to train their legs!

The solution

You can increase muscle mass in the leg area by concentrating on compound exercises, which cause maximum stimulation of the FT muscle fibres: squats, dead lifts and leg presses. These are, admittedly, harder to perform than isolation exercises such as leg extensions and curls (which should be avoided) as they require a great deal of physical and mental effort. However, they will produce faster and better results. Perform 3–4 sets per exercise for 6–10 repetitions, using heavy weights that allow you to reach failure.

Table 26.1	Symmetry programme for thin legs	
Exercise	**Sets**	**Reps**
Squat	3–4	6–10
Dead lift	3–4	6–10
Leg press	3–4	6–10

SYMMETRY PROBLEM: LACK OF HAMSTRING DEVELOPMENT RELATIVE TO QUADRICEPS

The back of your thigh appears straight and flat when viewed from the side as it is underdeveloped compared with the quadriceps. This imbalance is a common problem in long/middle-distance cyclists and runners as these activities stress the quadriceps more than the hamstrings. It is also seen in weight trainers who have concentrated on exercising the quadriceps and neglected to balance their leg programme with hamstring exercises.

The solution

The imbalance can be corrected by cutting back on quadriceps isolation exercises such as leg extensions, and by including more exercises for the hamstrings, such as leg curls and straight leg dead lifts. Use relatively heavy weights and keep the reps in the 6–10 range. All-round mass-builders such as squats and leg presses should still be included as they stimulate all the leg muscles equally.

Table 26.2	Symmetry programme for hamstrings	
Exercise	**Sets**	**Reps**
Squat or leg press	3–4	6–10
Straight leg dead lift	3–4	6–10
Lying or seated leg curl	3–4	6–10

SYMMETRY PROBLEM: FAT THIGHS

Fat thighs are more common in women than men, partly due to hormonal influences (oestrogen and progesterone favour fat deposition in the upper thighs and hips) and partly due to lifestyle. Eating more calories than you need and under-exercising over a period of time can cause an increase in body-fat stores. The only way to reduce fat is to combine increased aerobic exercise with a lower-calorie/-fat diet. Creams, massage, body brushes or 'detox' supplements cannot remove fat or cellulite.

The solution

The solution for fat thighs is to include both strength and aerobic (cardio) exercise in your programme, and reduce the fat content of your diet. Aim for a minimum of 20 minutes' cardio training 3–5 times a week, gradually increasing this to 45 minutes as you get fitter.

Table 26.3	Symmetry programme for fat thighs	
Exercise	**Sets**	**Reps**
Squat or leg press	2–3	12–15
Front or rear lunge	2–3	12–15
Lying or seated leg curl	2–3	12–15

SYMMETRY PROBLEM: SHAPELESS LEGS

Although you may have good strength in your legs, they may lack shape. Viewed from the front, your legs make a straight line from the hips to the knees, with no obvious outer sweep to the thigh. From the side, your legs also look straight and neither the quadriceps nor hamstrings make an aesthetic arc. This is due mainly to a lack of muscle development, a problem common among long-distance runners and people who exercise regularly but relatively infrequently (e.g. once a week).

The solution

Your programme should include a combination of compound exercises such as squats, and isolation exercises such as lunges and leg extensions to stimulate overall development. Use moderate to heavy weights and a mixture of low and high repetitions (8–15).

Table 26.4	Symmetry programme for shapeless legs	
Exercise	**Sets**	**Reps**
Squat or leg press	2	8–15
Front or rear lunge	2	8–15
Lying or seated leg curl	2	8–15
Leg extension	2	8–15

TRAINING FOR SPECIFIC RESULTS

SYMMETRY PROBLEM: SMALL CALVES

Small calves are partly due to genetics and partly due to lack of direct calf work. Some people have naturally thin calves due to a high percentage of ST fibres, so they have a low capacity for growth and are better suited to endurance work. It is a common mistake to neglect calf training, however. Many weight trainers leave them to the end of their workout, when they are tired, and perform little work on them.

The solution

If you have naturally thin calves you need to perform exercises that stress the small percentage of FT that you have there. Unfortunately, everyday activities such as walking and running work only the ST endurance fibres and provide minimal stimulation for growth. Therefore, your programme should include more emphasis on calf exercises. Perform 6–10 sets of 8–12 repetitions using heavy weights.

Table 26.5	Symmetry programme for small calves	
Exercise	**Sets**	**Reps**
Standing calf raise	2–4	8–12
Leg press machine calf-press	2–4	8–12
Dumbbell calf raise	2–4	8–12

SYMMETRY PROBLEM: BULKY CALVES

Bulky calves are usually due to the genetic endowment of a high percentage of FT fibres coupled with previous participation in sports such as sprinting, rugby, football and step aerobics. If you have a high percentage of FT fibres, your calves respond readily to any type of high-intensity exercise.

The solution

The only way to reduce the size of a muscle is to stop training it and allow it to atrophy (waste away). Realistically, you should minimise the amount of direct calf work you perform. They will receive sufficient stimulation from everyday activities, such as walking and running, your leg training and any sports that you play.

BACK CLINIC

SYMMETRY PROBLEM: NARROW BACK

Viewed from behind, your torso is straight, narrow and lacks a pleasing 'V' taper. This is mainly due to the underdevelopment of the back muscles and is a very common problem, especially in people who do little exercise. It is also seen in long-distance runners, joggers, cyclists, aerobics participants, and many other sportsmen, since relatively few sports and activities work this muscle group.

The solution

You can build and develop the muscles of the upper and mid back using heavy compound exercises, such as chins and rowing movements. Perform 3–4 sets of each exercise for 6–10 repetitions. The exercises in this programme build width and thickness.

Table 26.6	Symmetry programme for a narrow back	
Exercise	Sets	Reps
Chins	3–4	6–10
Bent-over barbell row or one arm row	3–4	6–10
Seated cable row	3–4	6–10

SYMMETRY PROBLEM: WEAK LOWER BACK

The muscles of your lower back, the spinal erectors, are easily overstretched and weakened through poor posture, bearing uneven and heavy loads, sudden twisting, poor exercise technique and lack of direct exercise. This leaves you prone to injury and back pain.

The solution

The lower-back muscles can be strengthened by specific exercises, but also by practising safe training techniques during exercises such as the squat and dead lift, which place considerable stress on this area. By holding the abdominals taut during these exercises – indeed during all exercises – you will help avoid injury and strain to the lower-back muscles. Include 3–4 sets of back extensions performed for 10–15 repetitions twice a week with your abdominal routine.

Table 26.7	Symmetry programme for a weak back	
Exercise	Sets	Reps
Back extension with Swiss ball	2–3	8–12
Crunch with Swiss ball	2–3	8–12

You should also strengthen your abdominal muscles – in particular, the deep (core) muscles in the abdomen and near the lower spine. Perform back extensions and abdominal exercises with the Swiss ball (exercise ball).

CHEST CLINIC

SYMMETRY PROBLEM: NARROW CHEST

A narrow chest has a straight appearance and makes the shoulders appear rounded and dominating. Viewed from the side it appears flat or even hollow. The width and circumference of your chest depends partly on your bone structure, in particular the size and shape of your ribcage and your clavicles (collarbones), and the size of your pectoral muscles.

The solution

A narrow chest can be improved by building up the pectorals and stretching the muscles between the ribs (serratus and intercostals). Poor posture can also exacerbate the symmetry problem, making the chest appear concave. This programme is

Table 26.8	Symmetry programme for a narrow chest	
Exercise	Sets	Reps
Barbell or dumbbell bench press (wide grip)	2–3	6–10
Incline barbell or dumbbell press	2–3	6–10
Dumbbell flye or cable cross-over	2–3	6–10

designed to develop the pectorals. You should use maximum ROM, particularly for the isolation exercises, and perform chest stretches between exercises to improve the flexibility of the pectorals and muscles of the ribcage. Perform 2–3 sets per exercise for 6–10 repetitions.

SYMMETRY PROBLEM: FLAT UPPER CHEST

Viewed from the side, the upper part of your chest appears flat or concave and lacks a pleasing aesthetic curve from your clavicles (collarbones). This symmetry problem is very common, particularly in women who have dieted, since the upper pectorals easily atrophy when calorie and protein intake is reduced over a period of time. A concave upper chest is due to underdevelopment of the upper portion of the pectorals.

The solution

Building the upper chest muscles corrects this problem and creates a fuller, more symmetrical chest. It also adds cleavage! Perform all pressing and flye movements on an incline bench set at 30–45 degrees. Use moderate–heavy weights, and perform 2–3 sets of 6–10 reps.

Table 26.9 Symmetry programme for a flat upper chest

Exercise	Sets	Reps
Incline bench press	2–3	6–10
Incline dumbbell press	2–3	6–10
Incline dumbbell flye	2–3	6–10

SHOULDER CLINIC

SYMMETRY PROBLEM: NARROW SHOULDERS

Narrow shoulders greatly affect your total body symmetry. In women, narrow, underdeveloped deltoids accentuate a pear shape, making the hips appear wider than they actually are. In men, they make the whole body look weak and undeveloped, or detract from an otherwise athletic physique. Sometimes, the medial (outer) head is poorly developed relative to the anterior (front) head. This is common in those weight trainers who focus on chest exercises such as the bench press at the expense of shoulder exercises.

The width of your shoulders is determined partly by the length of your clavicles (collarbones) and partly by the amount of muscle mass development. Obviously, you cannot change the former but you can significantly increase the width of your shoulders and greatly improve your overall body symmetry by developing your deltoids. The medial head is mostly responsible for creating width but all three heads need to be developed equally to create good symmetry and avoid injury.

The solution

To widen the shoulders, you need to build up the muscle mass by focusing on compound exercises such as shoulder presses and upright rows. These place the greatest stimulus on the shoulders and therefore lead to fastest gains in size and strength. You should also include lateral raises, as these work the medial head directly and create width. Perform 3–4 sets of 6–10 repetitions of each exercise, using heavy weights for the pressing movements.

Table 26.10	Symmetry programme for narrow shoulders	
Exercise	Sets	Reps
Dumbbell press	3–4	6–10
Upright row	3–4	6–10
Lateral raise	3–4	6–10

Table 26.11	Symmetry programme for rounded shoulders	
Exercise	Sets	Reps
Upright row	2–3	8–12
Bent-over lateral raise	2–3	8–12
Shrug	2–3	8–12
Shoulder press	2–3	8–12

SYMMETRY PROBLEM: ROUNDED SHOULDERS

Rounded shoulders are the result of poor posture, bad sitting position, poor muscle strength in the upper back and lack of flexibility in the chest muscles. Viewed from the side, your head juts forwards, your upper back is rounded, your ribcage is reduced, or even hollowed, and your shoulders droop. It is one of the most common postural faults in men and women. Rounded shoulders are also common in weight trainers who have overly developed the anterior head of the deltoids relative to the posterior head. Thus, the anterior head receives a disproportionate amount of stress compared with the medial and posterior heads, creating muscular imbalance.

The solution

Strengthening the trapezius and muscles of the upper back will pull the shoulders back into correct alignment. Increasing the flexibility of your chest muscles will expand the ribcage and allow the shoulders to move back easily into alignment. You should also strengthen the deltoids, especially the posterior head, which will help correct any muscular imbalance. Perform 3 sets of 8–12 repetitions of each exercise using a moderate weight.

ARM CLINIC

SYMMETRY PROBLEM: SKINNY ARMS

Poorly muscled arms are the result of a lack of direct biceps and triceps exercise. Your muscles are small and underdeveloped, lack density, appear straight and flat with no discernible shape.

The solution

The problem can easily be corrected by including mass-building exercises for your arm muscles, such as barbell curls, triceps extensions and triceps push-downs. These movements recruit the largest number of muscle fibres and therefore place maximum stress on the muscles, producing the fastest gains in size and strength.

Your programme should include more triceps work than biceps work because the triceps provide a much greater proportion of the upper-arm muscle mass than the biceps (see pp. 151–2). (Many weight trainers make the mistake of over-training their biceps and neglecting their triceps in an attempt to get bigger arms.) Select a total of 4–6 sets for your biceps, and 6–9 sets for your triceps, performing 6–10 repetitions per set with a heavy weight.

TRAINING FOR SPECIFIC RESULTS

Table 26.12	Symmetry programme for skinny arms		
Exercise		Sets	Reps
Barbell curl		2–3	6–10
Preacher curl		2–3	6–10
Lying triceps extension		2–3	6–10
Triceps press-down		2–3	6–10
Bench dip		2–3	6–10

Table 26.13	Symmetry programme for bulky arms		
Exercise		Sets	Reps
Concentration curl		2	10–15
Incline dumbbell curl		2	10–15
Dumbbell preacher curl		2	10–15
One arm triceps extension		2	10–15
Bench dip		2	10–15
Triceps kickback		2	10–15

SYMMETRY PROBLEM: BULKY, SHAPELESS ARMS

Viewed from the side, your arms appear chunky, straight and lacking in definition. You have developed good muscle mass but there is no real peak to the biceps, nor a discernible horseshoe outline to the triceps. This problem is partly due to excessive subcutaneous fat covering the muscles' outline, and partly due to poor exercise technique, shortening the ROM, which leads to sub-optimal development of the muscle along its whole length.

The solution

By reducing your body fat you will reduce the fat layer covering your triceps and biceps, and improve your muscle definition. So, include more cardio training (aim for 3–5 sessions of 20–30 minutes per week) and follow a fat-burning eating plan. The programme includes only one mass-building exercise for biceps and triceps, and two isolation exercises, which place greater demand on different parts of the muscles' length. Ensure that you use the full ROM and do not shorten the motion. Use slightly higher repetitions (up to 15) and moderate weights, and concentrate on the feel of the movement.

ABDOMINAL CLINIC

SYMMETRY PROBLEM: LOWER TUMMY BULGE

Viewed from the side, the lower part of your tummy appears rounded and protruding. This may be due to one or more of the following:

- poor posture
- poor muscle tone in the lower and deep abdominals
- overstretched abdominals
- an accumulation of fat.

The posture problem – lordosis – is caused by an excessive forward pelvic tilt. The hip flexors (which connect the thigh bone with the lower vertebrae) become tighter, and pull and compress the lower vertebrae, leading to excessive arching in your lower back.

The solution

Lordosis can be corrected by retraining the tilt of your pelvis (aim to maintain a neutral tilt), stretching the hip flexors and strengthening the abdominals (especially the lower part of the abdominis rectus and the transverse abdominis). Body fat should be reduced if necessary by increasing aerobic activity (aim for 3–5 cardio sessions per week of 20–45 minutes), and following a fat-burning eating plan. This programme emphasises the lower part of the rectus abdominis and the transverse abdominis, one of the deeper 'core' muscles (see p. 164) but also includes exercises for the other abdominal muscles to maintain good overall development. Performing the abdominal exercises using an exercise ball will strengthen the core muscles and improve stability (see p. 27).

Table 26.14	Symmetry programme for a lower tummy bulge	
Exercise	Sets	Reps
Reverse crunch	2	10–15
Hanging leg raise	2	10–15
Hip flexor stretch	2*	Hold for 30–60 seconds
Plank	1	Hold for 60–90 seconds
Exercise ball pull-in	1	10–15

*Perform twice on each leg.

SYMMETRY PROBLEM: WIDE WAIST

Viewed from the front, your waist appears wide relative to your hips and chest, and your tummy may protrude slightly. This may simply be due to a 'short' waist structure, or to an excess of fat stored at the sides of the waist and poor muscle tone of the obliques.

The solution

Fat stored at the sides of the waist cannot be spot-reduced by diet or exercise. However, it can be reduced when overall body-fat levels are reduced through increasing aerobic activity (3–5 cardio sessions per week of 20–45 minutes) and following a fat-burning eating plan.

Unfortunately, your basic skeletal structure cannot be changed. A naturally short midsection is determined by the distance between your ribs and pelvis, and can make the waist appear wider than it actually is. However, you can still improve your appearance by working the abdominal muscles and particularly the obliques. This will create a narrower waistline and better posture. This programme emphasises the internal and external obliques but also includes exercises for the rectus abdominis to maintain good overall development. Performing the abdominal exercises with an exercise ball will strengthen the core muscles, i.e. the deeper abdominal muscles and the muscles close to the lower spine and pelvis that improve your stability, coordination and posture.

Table 26.15	Symmetry programme for a wide waist	
Exercise	Sets	Reps
Oblique crunch	1–2	10–15
Side crunch	1–2	10–15
Alternate twisting	1–2	10–15
Swiss ball crunch	1–2	10–15
Side bridge	1–2	10–15

SUMMARY OF KEY POINTS

- Your personal training programme should be tailored to suit your natural body type, with a different emphasis placed on exercise selection, sets, repetitions, intensity and cardio training.
- Ectomorphs should focus on mass-building, using compound exercises, heavy weights, a high training intensity and limited cardio training.
- Endomorphs require more cardio training to burn fat, and can afford to do more sets and repetitions to increase calorie burning.
- Mesomorphs experience good gains from most programmes but should employ periodisation and plenty of variety to optimise developments and avoid overtraining.
- Your body-fat level depends on your genetic make-up, including your natural body type, as well as diet and activity.
- A body-fat percentage of 6–15 per cent for men and 10–20 per cent for women is generally associated with peak performance.
- A lower limit of 5 per cent body-fat for men and 14 per cent for women is recommended. Attaining lower body-fat percentages is associated with oestrogen deficiency in women and testosterone deficiency in men, as well as other health risks.
- Most symmetry problems can be remedied by using the SMART principles of programme design (see pp. 50–52) – selecting specific exercises, performed in a particular order for the right number of sets and repetitions, and at the correct intensity.

APPENDIX

Table App. 1	Quick reference for the major muscle groups, their locations, main functions and exercises		
Muscle	*Location*	*Main function*	*Exercises*
Legs Quadriceps • Rectus femoris • Vastus lateralis • Vastus medialis • Vastus interme- dius	Front of thigh	Collectively extend the knee. Rectus femoris also flexes the hip	Squat Dead lift Leg press Leg extension Front lunge Reverse lunge Dumbbell step-ups
Adductors • Adductor brevis • Adductor longus • Adductor magnus	Inner thigh	Pull the legs together	Squat Dead lift
Abductors • Gluteus minimus • Gluteus medius	Outer thigh	Pull the legs sideways	Squat Dead lift
Hamstrings • Biceps femoris • Semitendinosus • Semimembranosus	Back of thigh	Bend the knee and pull the hip back	Squat Dead lift Leg press Front lunge Reverse lunge Seated leg curl Straight leg dead lift Dumbbell step-ups

Muscle	Location	Main function	Exercises
Legs cont. Gastrocnemius	Calf	Bends the knee and straightens the ankle	Standing calf raise Single leg dumbbell calf raise Calf press Seated calf raise
Soleus	Calf	Straightens the ankle	Standing calf raise Single leg dumbbell calf raise Seated calf raise Calf press
Gluteals Gluteus maximus	Backside	Extends the hip and rotates it outwards	Squat Dead lift Leg press Front lunge Reverse lunge Straight leg dead lift Back extension Dumbbell step-ups
Gluteus medius	Backside	Abducts and rotates the hip inwards	Squat Dead lift Leg press Front lunge Reverse lunge Straight leg dead lift Back extension Dumbbell step-ups
Gluteus minimus	Backside	Stabilises the hip, and abducts and rotates it inwards	Squat Dead lift Leg press Front lunge Reverse lunge Straight leg dead lift Back extension Dumbbell step-ups

Muscle	Location	Main function	Exercises
Back			
Latissimus dorsi	Upper back	Draws the arms downwards	Dead lift Lat pull-down Pull-up/chin-up One arm dumbbell row Seated cable row Bent-over barbell row Straight arm pull-down Machine row Dumbbell pull-over
Trapezius	Upper and mid back	Draws the shoulder blades backwards	Dead lift Pull-up/chin-up One arm dumbbell row Seated cable row Bent-over barbell row Straight arm pull-down Machine row Dumbbell shrug *Dumbbell press* *Lateral raise* Upright row *Bent-over lateral raise*
Rhomboids	Deep central upper back	Draws the shoulder blades backwards	Lat pull-down Pull-up/chin-up One arm dumbbell row Seated cable row Bent-over barbell row Straight arm pull-down Machine row *Dumbbell press*
Infraspinatus	Shoulder blades	Rotates the arm outwards	Pull-up/chin-up One arm dumbbell row
Teres major	Shoulder blades	Rotates the arm outwards	Pull-up/chin-up One arm dumbbell row Seated cable row Bent-over barbell row Machine row Straight arm pull-down

Muscle	Location	Main function	Exercises
Back cont. Teres minor	Shoulder blades	Rotates the arm outwards	Pull-up/chin-up One arm dumbbell row Seated cable row Bent-over barbell row Straight arm pull-down Machine row
Erector spinae	Lower back	Flexes the spine and keeps you upright when standing	Barbell squat Dead lift Straight leg dead lift Back extension Back extensions Dorsal raise *Seated cable row*
Chest Pectoralis major	Chest	Pulls the arm in front of the chest from any position, flexes the shoulder to allow pushing and lifts the arm forwards	Barbell bench press Bench press machine Dumbbell bench press Dumbbell flye Pec-dec flye Cable cross-over Exercise ball press-up/push-up
Pectoralis minor	Chest	Lowers the shoulder blade	Incline barbell bench press Incline dumbbell bench press Low-pulley cable cross-over
Shoulders Anterior deltoids	Shoulder	Lift arm forwards and upwards	Dumbbell press Overhead press machine Upright row *Barbell bench press* *Dumbbell bench press* *Incline barbell bench press* *Incline dumbbell bench press* *Dumbbell flye* *Pec-deck flye* *Cable cross-over* *Lateral raise*
Medial deltoid	Shoulder	Lifts arm to the side	Dumbbell press Lateral raise Upright row Overhead press machine

Muscle	Location	Main function	Exercises
Shoulders cont. Posterior deltoid	Shoulder	Lifts arm to the rear and draws the elbow backwards	Bent-over lateral raise *Lat pull-down* *Chins* *One arm row*
Arms Triceps	Outside of the upper arm	Partially or fully straightens the arm from a bent position	Lying tricep extension Triceps kickback Triceps push-down Reverse-grip triceps push-down Seated overhead triceps extension *Barbell bench press* *Dumbbell bench press* *Incline barbell bench press* *Incline dumbbell bench press* *Dumbbell press* *Bench dip*
Biceps brachii	Front of the upper arm	Bends the elbow, rotates the forearm and assists in raising the shoulder forwards	Barbell curl Preacher curl Dumbbell curl Incline dumbbell curl Concentration curl *Lat pull-down* *Pull-up/chin-up* *One arm row* *Bent-over barbell row* *Upright row*
Brachialis	Front of the upper arm beneath the biceps	Bends the elbow	Barbell curl Preacher curl
Brachioradialis	Top side of forearm	Bends the elbow, rotates the forearm	*Lat pull-down* *Chins* *Seated cable row* *Bent-over barbell row* *Upright row*

Muscle	Location	Function	Exercises
Arms cont. Brachioradialis cont.			*Barbell curl* *Preacher curl* *Dumbbell curl* *Incline dumbbell curl* *Concentration curl* *Triceps push-down*
Abdominals Obliques – internal and external	Waist	Rotate and flex the trunk to the side	Side bridge Oblique crunch Side crunch Alternate twisting exercise-ball crunch
Rectus abdominis	Centre of the abdomen	Flexes the spine	Crunch Exercise ball crunch Reverse crunch Hanging leg raise Hip thrust Side crunch Exercise-ball pull-in Plank Side bridge Exercise-ball jackknife
Transversus abdominis	Sheathing the abdomen	Supports the abdomen	All the abdominal exercises performed with an exercise ball

Note: Exercises in italics indicate those in which the muscles are not the target muscles being developed.

REFERENCES

ACSM (2009), American College of Sports Medicine position stand. 'Progression models in resistance training for healthy adults'. *Med. Sci. Sp. Exerc.*, 41: 687–708.

Bacon A.P., Carter, R.E. Ogle, E.A. and Joyner, M.J. (2013), 'VO$_2$max trainability and high intensity interval training in humans: a meta-analysis', *PLoS NE* 8(9): e73182. <doi: 10.1371/journal.pone.0073182>

Baechle, T. R. and Earle, R.W. (eds) (2000), *Essentials of Strength Training and Conditioning*, Champaign, IL: Human Kinetics.

Baechle, T.R. and Groves, B. R. (1998), *Weight Training: Steps to Success*, 2nd ed. Champaign, IL: Human Kinetics.

Baker, S.K. *et al* (1994), 'Immediate post-training carbohydrate supplementation improves subsequent performance in trained cyclists', *Sports Med. Training Rehab.*, 5: 131–5.

Ballantyne, C.S., Phillips, S.M., MacDonald, J.R., Tarnopolsky, M.A., MacDougall, J.D. (2000), 'The acute effects of androstenedione supplementation in healthy young males', *Canadian Journal Of Applied Physiology*. 25(1): 68–78.

Balon, T. W. *et al* (1992), 'Effects of carbohydrate loading and weight lifting on muscle girth', *International Journal of Sport Nutrition*, 2: 328–4.

Bell, D.G. *et al* (2001), 'Effect of caffeine and ephedrine ingestion on anaerobic exercise performance', *Med. Sci. Sport Exerc.*, 33 (8): 1399–1403.

Bompa, T. O. and Cornacchia, L. J. (1998), *Serious Strength Training*, Champaign, IL: Human Kinetics.

Brilla, L.R. and Conte, V. (2000), 'Effects of a novel zinc-magnesium formulation on hormones and strength', *J. Exerc. Physiology.* 3(4): 1–15.

Broeder, C.E. *et al* (2000), 'The Andro Project', *Arch. Intern. Med.*, 160(20): 3093–104.

Brown, G.A. *et al* (1999), 'Effect of oral DHEA on serum testosterone and adaptations to resistance training in young men', *J. Appl. Physiol.*; 87: 2274–2283.

Brown, G.A. *et al* (2000), 'Effects of anabolic precursors on serum testosterone concentrations and adaptations to resistance training in young men', *International Journal of Sports Nutrition*, 10: 340–59.

Buford, T.W., *et al* (2007), 'International Society of Sports Nutrition position stand: creatine supplementation and exercise', *Journal of the*

International Society of Sports Nutrition, 4:6.

Burke, L.M. *et al* (2011), 'Carbohydrates for training and competition', *Journal of Sports Science*, 29(1): 17–27.

Burke, L.M. (2008) 'Caffeine and sports performance.' *Appl. Physiol. Nutr. Metab.*; 33(6): 1319–34.

Burke, L. (2007), *Practical Sports Nutrition.* Champaign, IL: Human Kinetics.

Campbell, W. *et al* (1994), 'Increased energy requirements and changes in body composition with resistance training in older adults', *Am. J. Clin Nutr.*, 60: 167–75.

Carter, J.M. *et al.* (2006), 'The effects of stability ball training on spinal stability in sedentary individuals,' *Journal of Strength Conditioning Research*, 20(2): 429-35.

Chowdhury, R. *et al.* 'Association of dietary, circulating and supplement fatty acids with coronary risk: a systematic review and meta-analysis', Annals of Internal Medicine online, <DOI: 10.7326/M13-1788>.

Churchward-Venne, T.A., Burd, N.A., Phillips, S.M. (2012), 'Nutritional regulation of muscle protein synthesis with resistance exercise: strategies to enhance anabolism', *Nutrition & Metabolism*, 9(1): 40.

Coffey, C.S., Steiner, D., Baker, B.A., Allison, D.B. (2004), 'A randomised double-blind placebo-controlled clinical trial of a product containing ephedrine, caffeine, and other ingredients from herbal sources for treatment of overweight and obesity in the absence of lifestyle treatment', *Int. J. Obes. Relat. Metab. Disord.*; 28(11): 1411–9.

Conley, M.S. and Stone, M. (1996), 'Carbohydrate ingestion/ supplementation for resistance exercise and training', *Sports Med.*, 21(1): 7–17.

Cooper, R. *et al* (2012), 'Creatine supplementation with specific view to exercise/sports performance (updated)', *Journal of the International Society of Sports Nutrition*, 9:33.

Cribb, P.J. and Hayes, A. (2006), 'Effects of supplement timing and resistance exercise on skeletal muscle hypertrophy', *Med. Sci. Sports Exerc.* 38(11): 1918–25.

Desbrow, B., *et al* 'Comparing the rehydration potential of different milk-based drinks to a carbohydrate-electrolyte beverage', *Appl Physiol. Nutr. Metab.* 14:1–7.

Doherty, M. and Smith, P.M. (2004), 'Effects of caffeine ingestion on exercise testing: a meta-analysis', *International Journal of Sports Nutrition and Exercise Metabolism.*, 14: 626–46.

Dons, B.K. *et al* (1979), 'The effect of weight lifting exercise related to muscle fibre composition and muscle cross-sectional area in humans', *Eur. J. Appl. Physiol.*, 40: 95–106.

Dorgan, J.F., *et al* (1996), 'Effects of dietary fat and fiber on plasma and urine androgens and estrogens in men: a controlled feeding study.' *Am. J. Clinical Nutrition*, 64(6): 850–5.

Draeger, C.L *et al* (2014), 'Controversies of antioxidant vitamins supplementation in exercise: ergogenic or ergolytic effects in humans?' *Journal of the International Society of Sports Nutrition*, 11: 4.

Drinkwater, E.J., *et al* (2007), 'Increased number of forced repetitions does not enhance strength development with resistance training', *Journal of Strength and Conditioning Research*, 21(3): 841–847.

Dulloo, A.G., *et al* (1999), 'Efficacy of a green tea extract rich in catechin polyphenols and caffeine in increasing 24 hour energy expenditure and fat oxidation in humans.' *Am. J. Clin. Nutr.* 70(6): 1040–5.

'Effect of a proprietary protein supplement on recovery indices following resistance exercise in strength/power athletes', (2010) *Amino Acids.* 38(3): 771-8. doi: 10.1007/s00726-009-0283-2. Epub 2009 Apr 4.

Elliot, T.A. *et al* (2006), 'Milk ingestion stimulates net muscle protein synthesis following restistance exercise,' *Med. Sci. Sports Exerc.*, 38(4): 667–74.

Evans, W. and Rosenberg, I. (1992), *Biomarkers*, New York: Simon & Schuster.

Fahey, T.D. *et al* (1993), 'The effects of intermittent liquid meal feeding on selected hormones and substrates during intense weight training', *Int. J. Sport Nutr.*, 3; 67–75.

Flack, K.D, *et al* (2011), Aging, resistance training, and diabetes prevention'. *Journal of Ageing Research.* 2011:127315.

Fleck, S.J. and Kraemer, W.J. (1997), *Designing Resistance Training Programmes*, Champaign, IL: Human Kinetics.

Forbes, G.B. (1976), 'The adult decline in lean body mass', *Human Biology*, 48: 161–73.

Forbes, S.C., Candow, D.G., Little, J.P., *et al*, 'Effect of Red Bull energy drink on repeated Wingate cycle performance and bench-press muscle endurance', *Int. J. Sport Nutr. Exerc. Metab.*, 17(5): 433–444.

Fortmann, S.P., Burda, B.U., Senger, C. *et al* (2013), 'Vitamin and mineral supplements in the primary prevention of cardiovascular disease and cancer: an updated systematic evidence review for the U.S. preventive services task force.' *Annals of Internal Medicine*, 159(12): 824–834.

Foster-Powell, K., Holt, S. & Brand-Miller, J. C. (2002), 'International table of glycaemic index and glycaemic load values', *Am. J. Clin. Nutr.*, 76; 5–56.

Friedl, K.E. *et al* (1994), 'Lower limit of body fat in healthy active men', *J. Appl. Physiol.*, 77: 933–40.

Gant, N., Ali, A., Foskett, A. (2010), 'The Influence of Caffeine and Carbohydrate Coingestion on Simulated Soccer Performance.' *Int. J. Sport Nutr. Exerc. Metab.*, 20: 191–197.

Garber, C.E., Blissmer, B., Deschenes, M.R., *et al* (2011): American College of Sports Medicine position stand. 'Quantity and quality of exercise for developing and maintaining cardiorespiratory, musculoskeletal, and neuromotor fitness in apparently healthy adults: guidance for prescribing exercise', *Medicine and Science in Sports Exercise*, 43(7): 1334–1359.

Garhammer, J. and McLaughlin, T. (1980), 'Power output as a function of load variation in Olympic and power lifting', Abstract: *J. Biomech.*, 13(2): 198.

Gleeson, M. (2008), 'Dosing and efficacy of glutamine supplementation in human exercise and sport training.' *J. Nutr.*, 138(10): 2045S–2049S.

Goldberg, A.L. *et al* (1975), 'Mechanism of work-induced hypertrophy of skeletal muscle', *Med. Sci. Sports Exerc.*, 7: 248–61.

Goldstein, E.R., Ziegenfuss, T., Kalman, D., *et al* (2010), 'International society of sports nutrition position stand: caffeine and performance', *J. Int. Soc. Sports Nut.* 7(1): 5.

Gualano, B., Roschel, H., Lancha-Jr, A.H., Brightbill, C.E., Rawson, E.S. (2012), 'In sickness and in health: the widespread application of creatine supplementation.' *Amino* Acids, 43: 519–529.

Halton, T.L. & Hu, F.B. (2004), 'The effects of high protein diets on thermogenesis, satiety and weight loss: a critical review.' *J. Am. Coll. Nutr.* 23(5): 373–85.

Hamalainen, E.K. *et al* (1983), 'Decrease of serum total and free testosterone during a low-fat high-fibre diet'. *J. Steroid Biochemistry*, 18(3): 369–70.

Harris, R.C., *et al* (2006), 'The absorption of orally supplied beta-alanine and its effect on muscle carnosine synthesis in human vastus lateralis.' *Amino Acids* 30(3): 279–89.

Hartman, J.W. *et al* (2007), 'Consumption of fat-free fluid milk after resistance exercise promotes greater lean mass accretion than does consumption of soy or carbohydrate in young, novice, male weightlifters.' *Am. J. Clin. Nutr.* 86: 373–381.

Holm, L.B. *et al* (2006), 'The effect of protein and carbohydrate supplementation on strength training outcome of rehabilitation in ACL patients.' *J. Orthop. Research.* 24: 2114–23.

Hartman, J.W., Tang, J.E., Wilkinson, S.B., Tarnopolsky, M.A., Lawrence, R.L., Hass, C.J. *et al* (2000), 'Single v. multiple sets in long-term recreational weightlifters', *Med. Sci. Sports & Exerc.*, 32(I): 235–42.

Hedrick, A. (1995), 'Training for hypertrophy', *Strength Cond.*, 17(3): 22–29.

Hobson, R.M., Saunders, B., Ball, G., Harris, R.C., Sale, C. (2012), 'Effects of β-alanine supplementation on exercise performance: a meta-analysis.' *Amino Acids.* 43(1): 25–37.

Hoffman J.R., *et al* (2010), 'Effect of a proprietary protein supplement on recovery indices following resistance exercise in strength/power athletes'. *Amino Acids*, 38(3): 771-8.

Hoon M.W., Hopkins, W.G., Jones, A.M., Martin, D.T., Halson, S.L., West, N.P., Johnson, N.A., Burke, L.M. (2014), 'Nitrate supplementation and high-intensity performance in competitive cyclists', *Applied Physiology, Nutrition, and Metabolism*, 0, 0, 10.1139/ apnm-2013-0574.

Hoon, M.W., Johnson, N.A., Chapman, P.G., & Burke, L.M., 'The effect of nitrate supplementation on exercise performance in healthy individuals: a systematic review and meta-analysis', *Int. J. Sport Nutrition, Exerc. Metab.* 23(5): 522-32. Epub 2013.

Houston, M.E. (1999). 'Gaining weight: The scientific basis of increasing skeletal muscle mass.' *Can. J. Appl. Physiol.*, 24: 305–316.

Hurley, B. (1994), 'Does strength training and muscle characteristics in untrained men improve health status?', *Strength & Cond. J.*, 16: 7–13.

International Olympic Committee (IOC) (2011), 'Consensus Statement on Sports Nutrition 2010', 4(29) Suppl 1:S3–4.

Ivy, J. L. *et al* (1988), 'Muscle glycogen synthesis after exercise: effect of time on carbohydrate ingestion', *J. Appl. Physiol.*, 64: 1480–5.

Jackman, S.R., Witard, O.C., Jeukendrup, A.E., Tipton, K.D. (2010), 'Branched chain amino acid ingestion can ameliorate soreness from eccentric exercise.' *Med. Sci. Sports Exerc.* 2(5): 962–70.

Karp J.R. *et al* (2006), 'Chocolate milk as a post-exercise recovery aid'. *Int. J. Sport. Nutr. Exer. Metab.* Feb; 16(1): 78–91.

King, D.S. *et al* (1999), 'Effects of oral androstenedione on serum testosterone and adaptations to resistance training in young men', J. Am. Med. Assoc., 281(21): 2020–8.

Kohrt, W, et al (2004), ACSM Position Stand: 'Physical Activity and Bone Health', Med. Sci. Sports Exer. 36(11): 1985–1996.

Koopman, R., (2005), 'Combined ingestion of protein and free leucine with carbohydrate increases postexercise muscle protein synthesis in vivo in male subjects.' Am. J. Physiol. Endocrinol. Metab. 288(4): E645–653.

Kraemer, W.J. et al (1995), 'Compatibility of high-intensity strength and endurance training on hormonal and skeletal muscle adaptations', J. Appl. Physiol., 78(3): 976–89.

Kreider, R.B. et al (2000), 'Effects of calcium-HMB supplementation during training on markers of catabolism, body composition, strength and sprint performance', J. Exerc. Physiol., 3(4): 48–59.

Lane A.R., Duke J.W., Hackney A.C. (2010), 'Influence of dietary carbohydrate intake on the free testosterone: cortisol ratio responses to short-term intensive exercise training', Eur. J. Appl. Physiol., 108(6): 1125–1131. <doi:10.1007/s00421-009-1220-5>.

Lane, S.C., et al (2014), 'Single and combined effects of beetroot juice and caffeine supplementation on cycling time trial performance', Appl. Physiol. Nutr. Metab. 39(9): 1050-7. <doi: 10.1139/apnm-2013-0336>. Epub 2013.

Lara, B., Gonzalez-Millán, C., Salinero, J.J. et al (2014), 'Caffeine-containing energy drink improves physical performance in female soccer players', Amino Acids, 46(5): 1385–1392.

Lemon, P.W.R. (1998), 'Effects of exercise on dietary protein requirements', Int. J. Sport Nutr., 8: 426–47.

Little, J.P., et al (2010), 'A practical model of low-volume high-intensity interval training induces mitochondrial biogenesis in human skeletal muscle: Potential mechanisms', The Journal of Physiology, 588(6): 1011.

Macdougall, J.D. et al (1979), 'Mitochondrial volume density in human skeletal muscle following heavy resistance training'. Med. Sci. Sports Exerc., 11(20): 164–6.

Macdougall, J.D. et al (1980), 'Muscle ultra-structure characteristics of elite powerlifters and bodybuilders'. Med. Sci. Sports Exerc., 2: 131.

Macdougall, J.D. et al (1994), 'Muscle fibre number in biceps brachii in bodybuilders and control subjects'. J. Appl. Physiol., 57: 1399–403.

Mackinnon, L.T., Hooper, S.L. (1996), 'Plasma glutamine and upper respiratory tract infection during intensified training in swimmers', Med. Sci. Sports Exerc. 28(3): 285–90.

MacLean, D.A., Graham, T.E., Saltin, B. (1994), 'Branch-chain amino acids augment ammonia metabolism while attenuating protein breakdown during exercise', Am. J. Physiol., 267, E1010–22.

Marcell, T.J. (2003), 'Sarcopenia: Causes, consequences, and preventions', J. Gerontol. A. Biol. Sci. Med. Sci. 58(10): M911–6.

McHugh, M.P., Cosgrave C.H. (2010), 'To stretch or not to stretch: the role of stretching in injury prevention and performance'. Scand. J. Med. Sci. Sports. 20(2): 169–81.

Menkes, A. et al (1993), 'Strength training increases regional bone mineral density and bone remodelling in middle-aged and older men' J. Appl. Physiol. 74: 2478–84.

MHRA (2012), 'MHRA warns public of potentially dangerous sports supplements': <http://

www.mhra.gov.uk/home/groups/comms-po/documents/news/con174847.pdf>

Moore, D.R., *et al* (2009), 'Ingested protein dose response of muscle and albumin protein synthesis after resistance exercise in young men,' *Am. J. Clin. Nutr.*, 89: 161–168.

Moraes, M.R., *et al.* (2012), 'Effect of 12 weeks of resistance exercise on post-exercise hypotension in stage 1 hypertensive individuals', *J. Hum. Hypertens*, 26(9): 533-9.

Neychev, V.K. and Mitev, V.I. (2005), 'The aphrodisiac herb Tribulus terrestris does not influence the androgen production in young men', *J. Ethnopharmacol*, 101(1–3): 319–2.

Ngo, T.H *et al* (2002), 'Effect of Diet and Exercise on Serum Insulin, IGF-I, and IGFBP-1 Levels and Growth of LNCaP Cells in vitro (United States)', *Cancer Causes & Control*, 3(10): 929–35.

Nielsen, F.H., Lukaski, H.C. (2006), 'Update on the relationship between magnesium and exercise', *Magnes. Res.*, 19(3): 180–9.

Nikolaidis, M.G., Kerksick, C.M., Lamprecht, M., McAnulty, S.R. (2012), 'Does vitamin C and E supplementation impair the favorable adaptations of regular exercise?', *Oxid. Med. Cell Longev.* 2012; 2012:707941. doi: 10.1155/2012/707941 (Epub 2012 Aug 13).

Nosaka, K., Sacco, P., Mawatari, K. (2006), 'Effects of amino acid supplementation on muscle soreness and damage', *Int. J. Sports Nutr. Exerc. Metab.*, 16: 620–635.

Osterberg, K.L. and Melby, C.L. (2000), 'Effect of acute resistance exercise on post-exercise oxygen consumption and resting metabolic rate in young women', *Int. J. Sport Nutr. Exerc. Metab.*, 10(1): 71–81.

Paddon-Jones, D. *et al* (2001), 'Short term HMB supplementation does not reduce symptoms of eccentric muscle damage', *Int. J. Sport Nutr.*, 11: 442–50.

Pasiakos, S.M., Cao, J.J., Margolis, L.M., *et al* (2013), 'Effects of high-protein diets on fat-free mass and muscle protein synthesis following weight loss: a randomized controlled trial', *FASEB Journal*, 27(9): 3837–3847.

Pasiakos, S.M., McClung, H.L., McClung, J.P. (2011), 'Leucine-enriched essential amino acid supplementation during moderate steady state exercise enhances postexercise muscle protein synthesis.' *Am. J. Clin. Nutr.* 94(3): 809–18.

Pasiakos, S.M., McClung, J.P. (2011), 'Supplemental dietary leucine and the skeletal muscle anabolic response to essential amino acids', *Nutr. Rev.* 69(9): 550–7.

Paulsen, G., Cumming, K.T. *et al* (2013), 'Vitamin C and E supplementation hampers cellular adaptation to endurance training in humans: a double-blind randomized controlled trial', *J. Physiol.* 2013: 267419.

Peternelj, T.T., Coombes, J.S. (2011), 'Antioxidant supplementation during exercise training: beneficial or detrimental?' *Sports Med.* 1,41(12): 1043–69.

Phillips, G.C. (2007), 'Glutamine: the nonessential amino acid for performance enhancement.' *Curr. Sports Med. Rep.* 6(4): 265–8. Review.

Phillips, S.M. (1996), 'Effect of training duration on substrate turnover and oxidation during exercise', *J. Appl. Physiol.*, 81(5): 2182–91.

Powers, M.E. (2002), 'The safety and efficacy of anabolic steroid precursors: What is the scientific evidence?' *J. Athletic Training*, 37(3): 300–5.

Phillips, S.M *et al* (2007), 'A critical examination of dietary protein requirements, benefits and excesses in athletes', *Int. J. Sports Nutr. Exerc. Metab.* 17: 58–78.

Phillips, S.M. and Van Loon, L.J. (2011), 'Dietary protein for athletes: from requirements to optimum adaptation' *J Sports Sci.*, 29(1): S29–38.

Quesnele, J.J., Laframboise, M.A., Wong, J.J., Kim, P., Wells, G.D. (2004), 'The effects of Beta-alanine supplementation on performance: a systematic review of the literature.' *Int. J. Sport Nutr. Exerc. Metab.* 24(1): 14–27.

Raastad, T., Bjøro, T., Hallén J., (2000) 'Hormonal responces to high- and moderate-intensity strength exercise', *Eur. J. Physiol.*, 82: 121-8.

Rawson, E.S., Volek, J.S. (2003), 'Effects of creatine supplementation and resistance training on muscle strength and weightlifting performance.' *J. Strength Cond. Res.*, 17: 822–831.

Risch, S. *et al* (1993), 'Lumbar strengthening in low back pain patients', *Spine*, 18: 232–8.

Rodriguez, N.R., Di Marco, N.M., Langley S.: American Dietetic Association; Dietitians of Canada; American College of Sports Medicine: American College of Sports Medicine position stand: 'Nutrition and athletic performance', *Med. Sci. Sports. Exerc.* 1(3): 709–31.

Rowlands, D.S., Thomson, J.S. (2009), 'Effects of beta-hydroxy-beta-methylbutyrate supplementation during resistance training on strength, body composition, and muscle damage in trained and untrained young men: a meta-analysis.' *J. Strength Cond. Res.* 23(3): 836–46.

Russell, C., Hall, D., Brown, P. (2013), European Supplement Contamination Survey, <www.informed-sport.com>.

Sale, C., Saunders B., Harris, R.C. (2010), 'Effect of beta-alanine supplementation on muscle carnosine concentrations and exercise performance.' *Amino Acids*, 39: 321–333.

Sale, D.G. *et al* (1987), 'Voluntary strength and women and bodybuilders', *J. Appl. Physiol.*, 62: 1786–93.

Schmidtbleicher, D. and Haralambie, G. (1981), 'Changes in contractile proteins of muscle after strength training in man', *Eur. J. Appl. Physiol.*, 46: 221–8.

Schwingshackl, L., *et al* (2013) 'Impact of different training modalities on anthropometric and metabolic characteristics in overweight/obese subjects: a systematic review and network meta-analysis'. *PLoS One.* 17(8): 12 <e82853. doi: 10.1371/journal.pone.0082853. eCollection 2013>

Sekendiz, B., Cuğ, M., Korkusuz, F. (2011), 'Effects of Swiss-ball core strength training on strength, endurance, flexibility, and balance in sedentary women.' *J. Strength Cond. Res.* 24(11): 3032-40.

Shimomura, Y., Inaguma, A., Watanabe, S. *et al* (2010), 'Branched-chain amino acid supplementation before squat exercise and delayed-onset muscle soreness.' *Int. J. Sport Nutr. Exerc. Metab.*; 20(3): 236–44.

Shirreffs, S.M., Watson, P., Maughan, R.J. (2007) 'Milk as an effective post-exercise rehydration drink.' *British Journal of Nutrition*, 1(8).

Shrier, I. (1999), 'Stretching before exercise does not reduce the risk of local muscle injury: a critical review of the clinical and basic science literature.' *Clin. J. Sport. Med.* 9(4): 221–7.

Shrier, I. and Gossal, K. (2000), 'Myths and truths of stretching', *Phys. Sportsmed.*, 28.

Slater, G., Jenkins, D., Logan, P., Lee, H., Vukovich, M., Rathmacher, J.A., Hahn, A.G. (2001), 'Beta-hydroxy-beta-methylbutyrate (HMB) supplementation does not affect changes in strength or body composition during resistance training in trained men', *Int. J. Sport Nutr.*, 11: 383–96.

Smith, J. and McNaughton, L. (1993), 'The effects of intensity of exercise and excess post-exercise oxygen consumption and energy expenditure in moderately trained men and women', *Eur. J. Appl. Physiol.*, 67: 420–5.

Stone M. et al (1999), 'Periodization: Effects Of Manipulating Volume And Intensity. Part 1' *Strength and Conditioning Journal*, 21(2): 56–62.

Stone, M. *et al* (1982), 'Physiological effects of a short-term resistance training programme on middle-aged untrained men', *Nat. Strength & Cond. Assoc. J.*, 4: 16–20.

Strauss, R.H. *et al* (1993), 'Decreased testosterone and libido with severe weight loss', *Phys. Sportsmed.*, 21(12): 64–71.

Taafe, D.R. et al (1997), 'High impact exercise promotes bone gain in well-trained female athletes', *J. Bone Miner. Res.*, 12(2): 255–60.

Tan, B. (1999), 'Manipulating resistance training program variables to optimise maximum strength in men', *J. Strength Cond. Research*, 13(3): 280–304.

Tarnopolsky, M.A. *et al* (1992), 'Evaluation of protein requirements for trained strength athletes', *J. Appl. Physiol.*, 73: 1986-95.

Tarnopolsky, M.A. *et al* (1997), 'Post exercise protein–carbohydrate and carbohydrate supplements increase muscle glycogen in males and females', *J. Appl. Physiol. Abstracts*, 4: 332A.

Tipton, K. & Wolfe, R. (2007), 'Protein needs and amino acids for athletes', *J Sports Sci*, 22(1): 65–79.

Tipton, K.D., Borsheim, E., Wolf, S.E., Sanford, A.P., Wolfe R.R. (2003), 'Acute response of net muscle protein balance reflects 24-h balance after exercise and amino acid ingestion'. *Am. J. Physiol. Endocrinol. Metab.*, 284(1): E76–89.

Tipton, K.D., et al (1999), 'Postexercise net protein synthesis in human muscle from orally administered amino acids'. *Am. J. Physiol.* 276(4,1): E628–34.

WADA (2014), 'The 2014 Prohibited List'. <www.wada-ama.org/en/ Science-Medicine/ Prohibited-List>.

Wang, Z., *et al* (2011), 'Evaluation of specific metabolic rates of major organs and tissues: Comparison between men and women'. *Am. J. Hum. Biol.*, 23: 333–338. <doi: 10.1002/ajhb.21137>

Weisgarber, *et al* (2012), 'Whey Protein Before and During Resistance Exercise Has No Effect on Muscle Mass and Strength in Untrained Young Adults'. *Int. J. Sport. Nutr. Exerc. Metab.* 22: 463-469.

Westcott, W.L. (2012), 'Resistance training is medicine: Effects of strength training on health'. *Curr Sports Med. Rep.* 11(4): 209Y16.

Wilborn, C.D., *et al* (2004), 'Effects of Zinc Magnesium Aspartate (ZMA) Supplementation on Training Adaptations and Markers of Anabolism and Catabolism.' *J. Int. Soc. Sports Nutr.* 1(2): 12–20.

Wilkinson, S.B *et al* (2007), 'Consumption of fluid skim milk promotes greater protein accretion after resistance exercise than does consumption of an isonitrogenous and isoenergetic soy-protein beverage,' *Am. J. Clin. Nutr.*, 85(4): 031–40.

Willardson, J.M. (2007), 'Core stability training: applications to sports conditioning programs, *J. Strength Cond. Res.* 3: 979-85.

Willis, L.H., Slentz, C.A., Bateman, L.A., *et al* (2012), 'Effects of Aerobic and/or Resistance Training on Body Mass and Fat Mass in Overweight or Obese Adults.' *J. Appl. Physiol.*, 15:113(12): 1831–7.

Willoughby, D.S. *et al* (2007), 'Effects of resistance training and protein plus amino acid supplementation on muscle anabolism, mass, and strength'. *Amino Acids*, 32(4): 467–477.

Wilson, J.M., *et al* (2013), 'International Society of Sports Nutrition Position Stand: beta-hydroxy-beta-methylbutyrate (HMB)' *J. Int. Soc. Sports Nutr.*; 10(1): 6.

Witvrouw, E, Mahieu N, Danneels L, McNair P. (2004), 'Stretching and injury prevention: an obscure relationship.' *Sports Med.* 2004; 34(7): 443–9.

Wolfe, R.R. (2006), 'The underappreciated role of muscle in health and disease'. *Am. J. Clin. Nutr.*, 84(3): 475–82.

Zawadski, K.M. *et al* (1992), 'Carbohydrate–protein complex increases the rate of muscle glycogen storage after exercise', *J. Appl. Physiol.*, 72(5): 1854–9.

FURTHER READING

Baechle, T.R. & Earle, R.W. (eds) (2008), *Essentials of Strength Training and Conditioning* (3rd ed.) Champaign, IL: Human Kinetics.

Baechle, T.R. & Groves, B.R. (2006), *Weight Training: Steps to Success* (3rd ed.) Champaign, IL: Human Kinetics.

Bean, A. (2013), *The Complete Guide to Sports Nutrition* (7th ed.) London: Bloomsbury Sport.

Bean, A. (2014), *Food for Fitness* (4th ed.) London: Bloomsbury Sport.

Bompa, T.O., Cornacchia, L.J. & Di Pasquale, M.G. (2002), *Serious Strength Training* (2nd ed.) Champaign, IL: Human Kinetics.

Fleck, S.J. & Kraemer, W.J. (2014), Designing Resistance Training Programmes (4th ed.) Champaign, IL: Human Kinetics.

King, I. & Schuler, L. (2003), *Men's Health: The Book of Muscle*, Rodale.

McArdle, W.D., Katch, F.I. and Katch, V.L. (2014), *Exercise Physiology: Nutrition, Energy and Human Performance* (8th ed.) Led & Febiger.

National Strength & Conditioning Association (2006), *Strength Training*, Champaign, IL: Human Kinetics.

Kenney, W.L., Wilmore, J.H. & Costill, D.L. (2011), *Physiology of Sport and Exercise* (5th ed.) Champaign, IL: Human Kinetics.

GLOSSARY

Actin A muscle protein that acts with myosin to produce muscular activity.

Aerobic In the presence of oxygen.

Agonist (prime mover) A muscle that is primarily responsible for bringing about a movement.

Alpha-linolenic acid An essential fatty acid, belonging to the omega-3 series.

Anabolic The building of body tissue.

Anaerobic In the absence of oxygen.

Antagonist The muscle that acts in opposition to the agonist, opposing the movement.

Atrophy The gradual wasting of a muscle.

Calorie A unit of energy measurement, defined as the amount of heat required to increase the temperature of 1 g of water by 1°C. The common unit used in food labelling is known as a kilocalorie (kcal) and has the value of 1000 calories.

Cardiovascular exercise ('cardio') Exercise that improves the efficiency of the cardiovascular (heart, blood and blood vessels) system.

Catabolic The breaking down of body tissue.

Compound, or multi-joint, exercise Involves one or more large muscle groups and works across two or more main joints.

Concentric The shortening of a muscle during contraction.

Descending (drop) sets A training method that involves performing repetitions to muscle failure followed immediately by further repetitions using a lighter weight until muscle failure is reached again.

Detraining The loss of fitness that occurs when you stop training

Eccentric The lengthening of a muscle under controlled tension.

Eccentric (negative) training Training that involves eccentric action.

Endurance The ability to resist fatigue.

Fast-twitch fibre A type of muscle fibre with a low aerobic capacity and high anaerobic capacity, which is best suited to speed and power activities.

Forced, or assisted rep, training A method of training that allows you to train past the point of muscular failure; a spotter provides assistance for the last 1 or 2 reps of a set.

Hypertrophy An increase in muscle size due to increased cell size.

Interval training Repeated brief high-intensity work interspersed with short periods of recovery.

Isolation, or single-joint, exercise For smaller groups of muscles and only one main joint.

Isometric A contraction where tension develops but there is no change in muscle length.

Ligament A strong band of fibrous tissue that connects bones to other bones.

Linoleic acid An essential fatty acid, belonging to the omega-6 series.

Macrocycle A period of training including several mesocycles, usually one season in duration.

Mesocycle A period of training usually 2–6 weeks long.

Microcycle A period of training, usually one week.

Motor unit The motor nerve and the group of muscles it innervates.

Muscle fibre An individual muscle cell.

Muscle spindles A sensory receptor in the muscle that senses how much the muscle is stretched.

Muscular failure An inability of the muscle to complete another repetition.

Myosin A muscle protein that acts together with actin to produce muscular contraction.

One-repetition maximum The maximum weight that can be lifted for one repetition.

Overload A training load that challenges the body's current level of fitness (e.g. strength) and has the scope to bring about improvements in fitness (e.g. strength).

Periodisation (training cycles) A process of structuring training into periods.

Power The ability to produce force and speed.

Pre-exhaustion training A method of training that involves performing an isolation exercise prior to the compound exercise to pre-exhaust the target muscle.

Prime mover (agonist) A muscle that is primarily responsible for bringing about a movement.

Progression A gradual increase of workload over a period of time.

Pyramid training A form of multiple-set training in which the weight is increased in each set and the number of repetitions reduced

Rating of perceived exertion A subjective assessment of how hard you are working.

Repetition One complete movement from the starting position to a position of maximum contraction and back to the starting position.

Set A group of repetitions.

Slow-twitch muscle A type of muscle fibre with a high aerobic capacity, low anaerobic capacity; best suited to endurance activities.

Strength The ability of a muscle to produce force.

Supersets Two or more sets of different exercises performed consecutively with no rest period.

Synergist A muscle that assists the agonists (prime movers) in bringing about a movement.

Tendons Bundles of collagen fibres that connect muscle to bone.

Toning A non-technical term that refers to a relative increase in strength, producing a firmer appearance and feel in the relaxed state.

Training intensity The quantitative element of training such as speed, strength or power.

Training volume The number of sets multiplied by the number of repetitions.

VO$_2$max (or maximum aerobic capacity) The maximum capacity for oxygen consumption by the body during maximal exertion.

INDEX

abdominal exercises 163
    cable rotation 179
    crunch 166
    exercise ball crunch 167
    exercise ball jackknife/pike 178
    exercise ball pull-in 175
    hanging leg raise 174
    hip thrust 172
    medicine ball twist 171
    oblique crunch 169
    plank 176
    reverse crunch 168
    roll-out (with exercise ball) 179
    side bridge/plank 177
    side crunch 173
    V-sits 170
abdominal muscles 164–5, 270
abdominal symmetry problems 262–3
advanced programme 223–9
agonist muscles 15
AKT 59
all or nothing principle 17
amenorrhoea 255
amino acids 67, 71, 88–9
antagonist muscles 15
anti-ageing 11
antioxidants 86

arm exercises 151
    barbell curl 153
    bench dip 159
    concentration curl 157
    dumbbell curl 155
    EZ-bar preacher curl 154
    incline dumbbell curl 156
    lying triceps extension 160
    preacher curl 154
    seated overhead triceps extension 162
    triceps kickback 161
    triceps push-down 158
arm muscles 151–2, 269–70
arm symmetry problems 261–2
assisted rep training 24–5
athlete's training programme 237–8
ATP (adenosine triphosphate) 90

back exercises *see* lower back exercises; upper back
    exercises
back muscles 120–1, 267–8
back strain 164
back symmetry problems
    narrow back 258–9
    weak lower back 259
balance trainers 28–9
beetroot juice 86–7
beginner's programme 210–16

beta-alanine 87–8
biological value (BV) 71
blood pressure 11
body fat 11, 13, 53, 77, 255
  see also fat loss
body types 20, 253–5
body weight exercises
  leg curl on exercise ball 180
  lunge twist 183
  plank variations 187–8
  push-up (close grip) 185
  push-up (feet elevated) 184
  side lunge 186
  single dead lift 180–1
  single leg bridge 188
  single leg split squat 182
  squat on BOSU ball 181–2
body weight workouts 232–3
bone density 11
Borg scale 248
BOSU balls 28–9
branched chain amino acids (BCAAs) 88–9,
  93–4
breathing 42

caffeine 89–90
calories 60–2
carbohydrates 63–7
  choice of 64–7
  glycaemic index (GI) 65–7
  loading 68
  requirement 63–4
  and weigh loss 78
cardiovascular exercise 79
cardiovascular programme 246–51
carnosine 87–8
catabolism 250
chest exercises 132
  barbell bench press 133–4
  cable cross-over 140

dumbbell flye 138
dumbbell press 135
  incline barbell bench press 136
  incline dumbbell bench press 137
  low-pulley cross-over 141
  pec-deck flye 139
  vertical bench press machine 134
chest muscles 132–3, 268
chest symmetry problems 259–60
cholesterol 11
citrus aurantium 91
Coleus forskohlii extract 91
compound exercises 36, 37
concentric muscle actions 15
coordination 19–20
core stability 27
core training 26–30
cortisol 70, 249
creatine 90–1
cyclist's training programme 243

dehydration 69
descending (drop) sets 25, 224–5
detraining 40
dynamic stretching 203

eccentric muscle actions 15
eccentric training 24
ectomorphs 20, 253–4
endomorphs 20, 253–4
endurance, muscular 14, 31, 39
ephedrine 91
essential fatty acids 73
excess post-exercise oxygen consumption
  (EPOC) 246–7, 248
Exercise Register 55
exercise (stability) balls 27–8

fast-twitch muscle fibres 16–17, 19, 20, 25
fat burners 91

fat-burning zone myth 248
fat loss 11, 31, 62, 75, 78, 248
fats 11, 71–4, 78
fibre 79
flexibility 13, 201
food diaries 79
footballer's training programme 239
forced rep training 24–5
free radicals 86
free weights 48–9
full-body routines 39–40

glucose 63, 64, 65, 69, 75
glutamine 91–2
gluteal muscles 106, 266
glycaemic index (GI) 65–7
glycogen 63
goal-setting 45, 50–2
golgi tendon organs (GTOs) 201
green tea extract 91
growth hormone (GH) 21
GTO threshold 202
gyms 46–8

heart rate 247–8
high-calorie snacks 77
high-intensity interval training (HIIT) 248–9
hip flexors 106
HMB (beta-hydroxy beta-methylbutyrate) 92–3
home gyms 46, 47
hormonal balance 21
hydration 96
hyperplasia 19
hypertrophy 18–19, 25, 34, 39

injury prevention 12
insulin 63
intermediate's programme 217–22
interval training 248–9, 250

isolation exercises 36, 37
isometric muscle actions 15

joints 13

kinesthetic awareness 29
knee wraps 50

leg exercises see lower body exercises
leg muscles 104–6, 265–6
leg symmetry problems 256–8
ligaments 10
lordosis 164, 262
lower back exercises 120
    back extension on bench 130
    back extension on exercise ball 131
    back extension on floor 130
    Superman 131
lower body exercises 104
    calf (or toe) press 119
    dead lift 110
    dumbbell single leg calf raise 118
    dumbbell step-ups 115
    front lunge 113
    front squat 108
    leg extension 112
    leg press 111
    lunges 113–15
    reverse lunge 113–14
    seated leg curl 115
    Smith machine squats 108
    split squat 109–10
    squats 107–10
    standing calf raise 117
    straight leg dead lift 116
    walking lunge 114–15
lower body muscles
    gluteals 106
    hip flexors 106
    legs 104–6

INDEX

285

low-intensity cardiovascular exercise 248, 249

machines 49
martial artist's training programme 244
maximum heart rate (MHR) 247
maximum strength 38
meal planning 79–83
meal replacement products 88
measurements logs 53–4
mesomorphs 20, 253–5
metabolic rate 10–11, 61
methylhexaneamine (DMAA) 91
minerals 94
monounsaturated fats 73
motivation 52–5
motor units 21
mTOR (Mammalian Target of Rapamycin) 59
multivitamins 94–5
muscle fibres 16–17, 19, 20, 25
muscle gain menu plans 79–83
muscle groups 265–70
  abdominals 164–5, 270
  arms 151–2, 269–70
  back 120–1, 267–8
  chest 132–3, 268
  gluteals 106, 266
  legs 104–6, 265–6
  shoulders 142–3, 268–9
muscle imbalance 202
muscle mass 10
muscle protein breakdown (MPB) 59
muscle protein synthesis (MPS) 59
muscle(s) 102–3
  actions 15
  contraction 18
  fitness 14
  growth 18–20
  mass 20–1
  size 32–3, 39
  structure 15–16

muscle spindles 201
muscle tone 20

negatives 24
neuromuscular adaptation 19
neutral posture 27
nitrates 86
nitric oxide (NO) 86–7
nutrition
  calories 60–2
  carbohydrates 63–7, 78
  fats 71–4, 78
  for muscle gain 79–83
  nutrient timing 74–5
  protein 67–71, 78–9
  and recovery 41
  supplements 85–99
  for weight gain 75–7
  for weight loss 78–9

oestrogen 95, 255
omega-3 fatty acids 73, 74
omega-6 fatty acids 73–4
one-rep max (IRM) 23
overload 19, 25, 43, 223
  see also progressive training

partners, training 53
periodisation 30–4
personal appearance 12
personal trainers 54–5
phosphocreatine (PC) 90
Pilates 27
polyunsaturated fats 73
posture 12
post-workout snacks 76
power 14, 38–9
power/plyometric exercises
  box jump 193
  bunny hops 192

STRENGTH TRAINING

burpees 189
chest throw with medicine ball 195
clean and jerk 199
mountain climbers 191
plyo push-ups 191
power clean 198
seated overhead throw 196
snatch 200
split squat jumps 190
squat jumps 190
standing throw to floor 197
vertical depth jump 194
power/plyometric workouts 234–5
pre-exhaustion training 26, 37, 228–9
prime mover muscles 15
progesterone 255
programme design 36–45
exercise order 37–8
exercise selection 36
proper technique 41–2
rest periods 40–1
sets and reps 38–40
specificity 37
training intensity 40
troubleshooting 42–5
progressive training 23–6
prohormones 95
proprioception 29
protein 67–71, 78–9
psychological well-being 12
pumped, getting 26
pyramid training 24

range of motion (ROM) 13, 44
rate of perceived exertion (RPE) 249
record keeping 53–4
recovery drinks 95–6
rehydration 96
resistance bands 29–30
resistance training 250

rest 43
resting metabolic rate (RMR) 10–11, 61
rewards 55
rugby player's training programme 241–2
runner's training programme 242

saturated fats 72–3
sets and reps 23, 38–40
shoulder exercises 142
barbell shoulder press 145
bent-over lateral raise 150
dumbbell shoulder press 144
front lateral raise 148
lateral raise 147
overhead press machine 146
upright row 149
shoulder muscles 142–3, 268–9
shoulder symmetry problems 260–1
sit-up controversy 165
size principle 17
sliding filament theory 18
slow-twitch muscle fibres 16–17, 20, 25
SMART goals 50–2
specificity 37
speed of lifting 40
split workouts 39–40
sports-specific training 236–45
sprinter's training programme 237–8
starvation adaptation response 62
static stretching 203
steady pace training 248
stimulants 91
straps 49–50
strength 10, 14, 34, 38
strength programme 230–1
strength training myths 12–13
stretches
adductor 204
calf 205
chest/biceps 207

INDEX

hip flexor 204
hips/gluteal/outer thigh 204
lower back 205
lying glute 205
shoulder 206
standing quadriceps 203
triceps 207
upper back 206
stretching 57, 201–3
supersets 25–6, 38, 226–7
supplements 85–99
antioxidants 86
beetroot juice 86–7
beta-alanine 87–8
branched chain amino acids 88–9, 93–4
caffeine 89–90
creatine 90–1
fat burners 91
glutamine 91–2
HMB (beta-hydroxy beta-methylbutyrate) 92–3
leucine 93–4
multivitamins 94–5
prohormones 95
recovery drinks 95–6
stimulants 91
testosterone boosters 96–7
whey protein 97–8
ZMA 98–9
swimmer's training programme 240
synergist muscles 16

target heart rate zone (THR) 247
technique 41–2, 44
tendons 10, 201
tennis player's training programme 245
testosterone 21, 71, 95, 98, 104
testosterone boosters 96–7
training belts 49
training gloves 49

training to failure 24
triglycerides *see* fats
troubleshooting 42–5
goal-setting avoidance 45
lack of progression 43–4
not enough rest 43
partial range of movement 44
poor technique 44
too many reps 43
too many sets 43
wrong exercises 43

upper back exercises 120
bent-over barbell row 126
dumbbell pull over 128
dumbbell shrug 129
lat pull-down 122–3
machine row 127–8
one arm dumbbell row 124
pull-up/chin-up 123
seated cable row 125
straight arm pull-down 127

variety 54
visualisation 52
vitamins 94–5

warming up 56–7
weight gain 21, 75–7
weight loss 78–9
see also fat loss
well-being 12
whey protein 97–8

yohimbine 91

ZMA (zinc and magnesium aspartate) 98–9